Jane Scrivner's

TOTAL
DETOX

Other books by Jane Scrivner

Detox Yourself

Detox Your Mind

Detox Your Life

The Litte Book of Detox

Jane Scrivner's
TOTAL
DETOX

6 WAYS TO REVITALISE YOUR LIFE

PIATKUS

To Kevin as ever, thanks m'dear.

Copyright © 2000 by Jane Scrivner

First published in 2000 by
Judy Piatkus (Publishers) Limited
5 Windmill Street
London W1T 2JA
e-mail: info@piatkus.co.uk

For the latest news and information on all our titles,
visit our website at www.piatkus.co.uk

A catalogue record for this book is available from the British Library

ISBN 0 7499 2153 6

Edited by Kelly Davis
Design by Zena Flax

This book has been printed on paper manufactured with respect for the
environment using wood from managed sustainable resources

Data manipulation by Phoenix Photosetting, Chatham, Kent
Printed and bound in Great Britain by The Bath Press, Somerset

Contents

Introduction

Total Detox takes into account every aspect of detox. You can detox your mind, body, spirit and environment. You can detox for very important health reasons or you can detox just to change one particular aspect of your life. You can detox for the whole of your life, or pinpoint some key areas that need specific cleansing and revitalisation. You can totally detox for a full 30 days or you can dip your toe in the water and detox for just a few days. Every approach will have startlingly pleasing results and every approach has the potential to change your life in a positive way for ever.

If you have ever woken up feeling that:

- Everything needs to change . . .
- You need a fresh outlook . . .
- You need to clear the fuzz in your head . . .
- You need to clear the over-indulgence from your body and mind . . .

- You want to spend a few days looking after number one . . .
- Your home needs cleaning and your space needs cleansing . . .
- You need to wash that man/woman right out of your hair . . .
- You are doing the same old thing every day . . .

Then detox is just what you need. Everything can be done at home if you wish, at little or no expense. All it takes is you, and your desire to make life just a bit better. Alternatively, you can explore new treatments and experiences outside your home – a little investment can make a big difference.

Total Detox includes full programmes for yourself, your mind, your body, your life. *Total Detox* will show you how to make a difference – in just a weekend or in the full 30 days.

There are many ways to detox, and *Total Detox* will take you through practical, no nonsense, easy-to-achieve steps to make you feel better than ever. We don't ask you to grow beans on your windowsill, totally redecorate your flat in fuschia pink or change your career. We realise that your life is already busy and full. We just give simple, plain instructions that have massive, world-beating results. Sometimes we may tell you things you already know. Congratulations! You have already started to look at your own life and been made aware of how to look after yourself better and more effectively. It is always worth hearing good advice more than once. Who knows – you may just start to take it!

There are sections to show you just what a difference a day makes – well, 48 hours to be precise. By making some simple changes over just two days you can make the world of difference. Forget the bikini diets. Detox for a weekend and you get a flatter stomach than you could ever dream of, clearer skin, a more positive outlook and a 'well done' to yourself for being so good. *Total Detox* will take you from the negative to the positive and eliminate the bad to make room for the good – so what are you waiting for . . .?

THE TOTAL DETOX PROGRAMMES

PROGRAMME 1: THE 30-DAY ULTIMATE DETOX

A 30-day programme (p. 8) to cleanse your system of all toxins and waste and boost your immunity to promote full and flourishing health. A programme to make you feel better after a long period of overdoing it or simply to balance your diet and flush out your system. The Ultimate Detox looks at mind and spirit as well as body. It covers every aspect of your life, inside and out, physical and emotional. No stone is left unturned and every aspect is left improved and ready to go. This is a thorough detox programme to create a new, refreshed, re-energised and revitalised you.

PROGRAMME 2: THE QUICK-FIX HANGOVER DETOX

For those times when you have just too good a time and end up over-doing it. This programme (p. 56) has some handy hints on ways to prepare for partying and how best to spend the morning and day after. Supplements, exercise and attitude will help you to get you through the over-indulgence and apologise to your body for the abuse. There are also ways to prevent anything like that happening again – the 'never again' solutions.

This programme is not for the faint-hearted but the results are simply amazing and totally worth the effort. It's healthy to be realistic about the fact that we 'overcook' our lives once in a while, and finding ways to make it less damaging is even healthier.

PROGRAMME 3: THE HEALTHY MIND DETOX

It is not enough to have a healthy body if you are not thinking straight or feeling good about yourself. Keep your mind active and develop a new view of your life, develop enough self-esteem and confidence to go out and get just what you want. Drag yourself out of the doldrums or simply boost your positive energy.

This is a 10-day programme (p. 64) to get you looking at things in a different light. If you're feeling stubborn or you don't seem to be able to get on with life then a quick reassessment may just change the way you feel. If things are not going your way maybe looking at them from a different angle could give you the answers you need.

The Healthy Mind Detox will bring a smile to your face and a feel-good factor into your life.

PROGRAMME 4: THE WEEKEND DETOX

For those rare times when you find you have 48 hours to concentrate on number one. Lock the doors, put the ansaphone on and switch off the mobile. This two-day plan (p. 90) will transform you from a tired and worn-out 'human doing' on Friday afternoon to a revitalised, refreshed and regenerated 'human being' on Monday morning. Create your own home spa with the Weekend Detox and you will feel amazing: slough your way to svelte, smooth limbs and streamline yourself to sleek, toned slenderness. Detox can be pure indulgence – no, really – massage, aromatherapy, exfoliation, wraps and rubs. All these can purge you of unwanted toxins and promote internal healing and external fabulousness!

Enrol some friends but make sure you are totally dedicated to the stunning new you. No one else matters. This is your time to make *you* feel great.

PROGRAMME 5: THE COMPLETE HOME DETOX

Feng Shui the fug and clear the clutter, or just spring-clean the cupboards and wipe the ketchup bottle! Give your home a makeover and feel the benefit of getting things in the right place and looking after your space. Welcome the good ghosts and banish the bad vibes – live in peace and harmony and let your surroundings work for you.

This five-point plan (p. 129) will change the way you live and add some colour and sparkle to your home and surroundings. The Complete Home Detox can also work wonders at work. Try the plan with your colleagues or friends and see how good it feels to get things sorted. Small changes can have huge effects. If you have ever had doubts about the colour, shape or position of a piece of furniture then now is the time to move it, turn it round or get rid of it altogether.

PROGRAMME 6: THE RELATIONSHIP DETOX

Partners, friends and family all play an incredibly important part in our lives. Sometimes they make you happy and sometimes they drive you bananas. You can spend time with someone and feel fabulous or just have a short phone conversation with a regular friend that will make you want to scream. The Relationship Detox (p. 146) gets you to look at your relationships and see how to get the best out of them, how to boost them and how to know when to leave them alone for a while. Our relationship with ourselves is also incredibly important – until we start treating our self, respecting our self and boosting our self, we cannot expect to be able to do all these things for anyone else. If we are fulfilled than we can give; if we are drained and tired then we need to boost ourselves back up to full strength. The Relationship Detox will give you all the support you need to do this.

Detoxing is a big decision. You are deciding to change your life for the better, to take some steps that will improve the way you feel both inside and out. You will be noticeably different to friends and family but, most importantly, you will be different to yourself. You will have taken your life into your own hands and taken full responsibility for getting to where you want to be. It won't be easy but the benefits will far outweigh the efforts. Just knowing you can change yourself or your life is pretty amazing, and achieving it is even better.

Important Note

You should not start any of the programmes if any of the following applies to you at the time of your detox:

- If you are pregnant.

- If you are breast-feeding.

- If you are undergoing medical treatment for any illness or condition.

- If you are recovering from a serious illness.

- If you are taking any prescribed or non-prescribed drugs.

- If you have any doubts about your own well-being.

- If your doctor has advised you against changing your diet or has put you on a specific diet.

Within this book there is something for absolutely everyone at absolutely any time. The programmes can all be carried out on a normal day-to-day basis – there's no need to take a month off work or make any special arrangements. All you need is the desire to make things better for yourself, a little preparation and a little application – the results are simply amazing and the effort totally worthwhile.

THREE KEY POINTS

- Each programme needs a little preparation to make it easier to follow. There is a list at the start of the sections where pre-preparation is required – follow this list and you will have already detoxed some clutter from your mind.

- Each programme has some extra 'in-depth' details if you wish to access them. These details can be found in the User's Manual at the back of the book. Everything you need to know in order to get the best out of the programmes is contained in this section. For example, look here for information on breathing techniques, where to get the best advice on booking a Feng Shui consultation, or the full ingredients list for a recipe for the 48-hour detox evening in. Nothing is left to chance.

- Each programme needs your fully co-operative open mind and your willingness to learn. Read on, choose a programme that is most appropriate to your needs, or alternatively just work through them all one by one.

Good luck and thank you. What are you waiting for!

1 The 30-Day Ultimate Detox

The Ultimate Detox is not just about food; you will be doing some fun, strange, odd and exciting things for your mind, body and spirit. Make sure that you really *do* want to make the changes, then truly commit to the new you.

PREPARING FOR YOUR ULTIMATE DETOX

In order to get the best out of your 30-Day Ultimate Detox you need to take some preliminary steps so that nothing dissuades you from your goal and nothing stops you once you have started.

Where you are now determines how and when you start your Ultimate Detox programme. If you live on toxins, eat only fast food and constantly live on the edge, then we have some work to do. If you just need to formalise your already healthy way of life some interesting changes and more effective moves then you are just moments away from your own personal programme.

Also, as we've already established, there are a few rules that absolutely must be observed. Most importantly, you should not be starting a detox if you are ill, pregnant or breast-feeding. It is unlikely to cause any damage but it will mean asking your body to work hard at a time when it is already working hard enough. It is best to wait until you are back to your normal state of health and harbouring no germs or viruses. If you are pregnant, wait until you have had your baby and have finished breast-feeding.

ULTIMATE DETOX SELF-ASSESSMENT

Once you have established that you are ready for the Ultimate Detox, then you can begin. By answering some simple questions you can find out if you are already on the starter's block or if you need to do a few days' preparation before launching into the full programme.

For each question, tick the answer that best describes your current situation:

1 How do you rate your current diet?

Very healthy   ☐   (3 points)
Fairly healthy   ☐   (2 points)
Bad   ☐   (1 point)

2 How are your energy levels?

Good   ☐   (3 points)
OK   ☐   (2 points)
Low   ☐   (1 point)

3 Which best describes your activity levels?

Regular exercise and/or an active job or life ☐ (3 points)

Some exercise but a sedentary job ☐ (2 points)

No exercise and a sedentary job ☐ (1 point)

4 How much water do you drink per day?

1.5 litres (3 pints) ☐ (3 points)

3–4 glasses ☐ (2 points)

Less than 3 glasses ☐ (1 point)

5 How much coffee, tea or canned drinks (Cola etc) per day?

Few or none ☐ (3 points)

About three ☐ (2 points)

Six or more ☐ (1 point)

6 How much alcohol do you drink per week?

4–6 units ☐ (3 points)

8–12 units ☐ (2 points)

15 units or more ☐ (1 point)

7 How much fresh fruit or vegetables do you eat every day?

3–4 portions ☐ (3 points)

1–2 portions ☐ (2 points)

1 or none ☐ (1 point)

Now add your scores together and read your assessment below:

Scores above 14

If you scored above 14 you should be able to start the Ultimate Detox without any further preparation. Well done and good luck!

Scores below 14

If you scored below 14 you should consider making some preliminary changes before starting your Ultimate Detox. These changes should help smooth your transition into the programme and prevent those niggling headaches and side-effects from detoxing.

Try to implement these changes at least 10 days before commencing the Ultimate Detox programme.

Things to do if your score was below 14:

- Start doing some mild exercise, a walk at lunchtime or running up and down the stairs five times before bed – anything that will increase your pulse rate for 20 minutes each day.

- Make sure you drink at least 1.5 litres (3 pints) of water a day.

- Halve your alcohol intake.

- Halve your coffee, tea and fizzy drink intake.

- Make sure you eat at least 3 portions of fruit each day. (1 portion of fruit is an apple or a pear, etc.)

- Make sure you eat at least 3 portions of vegetables each day. (1 portion of vegetables is one large serving spoon or more.)

- Reduce your intake of bread and pasta to 1 portion per day.

Now you are ready to pull your body, mind and spirit back from the brink of over-toxing . . .

A FEW MORE PREPARATION TIPS

Choose your time carefully

The Ultimate Detox lasts for 30 days. During this time you will follow a day-by-day programme that will finish in the new you. It will not be easy but it will be a wonderful experience. You should choose a time when you can enjoy the programme to its full.

January and February are good. The recovery period after Christmas is a great time for taking stock, cleansing through your body, making life decisions and saving money! Depending on when Easter falls, February, March or April are good candidates, there are plenty of fruits and vegetables around and spring is a season of new beginnings and fresh starts. Just avoid the Easter break if you know that chocolate will be too much of a temptation.

If you are planning a holiday to a retreat or health farm then that is a great time to commence the programme. But if your vacation is two weeks with 15 friends in Ibiza it might be best to wait until after the holiday.

If your social diary is full then wait until you have a space of at least two weeks. This will give you a chance to get used to the new plan and go through any initial changes without having to constantly turn down offers of sandwiches, alcohol or coffee mornings that may prove too tempting.

Think about all these factors and consult your diary. Find the best time and if it is not in the next few days then that's OK. It's often the case that the thing most waited for, is the thing best received.

Be positive

Once you have named the day, you can start to prepare your friends. There is something very tempting about trying to break down someone's new resolve, ruin their good intentions or persuade them that they couldn't possibly achieve their new goals. Your own human nature will be addressed in the programme but you also need to prepare for everybody else's.

When you explain the programme to friends, don't tell them how different it is from normal and how time-consuming it is to get everything done. Instead, tell them how many positive changes you have made and how you are doing much more every day due to your increased energy levels and your enthusiastic state of mind. Enjoying the programme and letting your friends know just how great you are feeling and how positively you are thinking will get them curious and supportive from the moment you start.

Think of the Ultimate Detox programme as you own personal month at a health farm. You should enjoy each day of the programme. Don't always think about how long you have to go but think about how much you have already done and how good you are feeling. Most people have now heard of the principle of detoxing but many still don't know what it is or aren't prepared to make the changes to their own life. When you tell people what you are doing they will be very interested. You may even find that you enrol a fellow detox mate so that you have a friend to call on when you want to compare menu ideas or discuss where to get a good facial.

PREPARATION LISTS

There are some things that you need to gather or source so that you have them ready for when you start. Many of these you will already have, or will know where to get hold of, but you should do this in plenty of time. Having them ready makes the programme go smoothly and a little preparation is never a bad thing.

CHECK LIST OF ESSENTIALS

- **Airtight food containers** Tupperware, for example.

- **Steamer** Metal or bamboo (the type you put over or in a pan of hot water to steam vegetables or fish).

- **Skin brush** Natural bristles. The bristles should be firm but not too stiff, otherwise they may irritate your skin.

- **Exfoliating creams or salt** Use up odds and ends of creams to save money. If they are not exfoliants add a teaspoon of salt or sand and this will do the job.

- **Loofah or flannel mitt** Use a towelling or natural fibre mitt.

- **Somewhere to exercise** Gym, bedroom, stairs, lounge, etc.

- **Bath or shower** Access to both a bath and shower is ideal but one or the other is fine.

Check list of optional/luxury items

- **A juicer** This is a definite luxury but what better time to try making your own juice than during the Ultimate Detox?

- **Organic foods** There are many suppliers of organic fruit, vegetables and fish prepared to deliver nationally (see Useful Addresses). Alternatively, many supermarkets now stock organic produce which is fortunately not too much more expensive than regular produce. But beware of the food going off quickly. The secret with organic food is to buy little and often. Using organic foods will automatically reduce your intake of pesticides (which are routinely sprayed on most conventionally grown fruit and vegetables). Organic foods are not essential – the fact that you are actually going to be eating fresh foods over the next month is probably enough of a change. But if fruit and vegetables already form the basis of your diet then try organics and see if you notice a difference.

SHOPPING LIST

There are some more unusual items – on top of your meals – that you will be required to eat or drink every day and these should be bought in advance as you are unlikely to have them in stock. Some may sound a bit odd but all will be revealed!

- **Vegetable juice** Bottled carrot or beetroot juice is usually available from your local healthfood shop. Start with one bottle. Alternatively, if you have a juicer, buy fresh vegetables and juice your own.

- **Olive oil** Try to buy extra-virgin, cold-pressed or first-pressed oils as these are purer. They are available in all supermarkets – 1 litre (2 pints) will do to start.

- **Fresh garlic and odourless garlic pills** From greengrocers and healthfood shops – buy enough pills for one a day or a large bulb to start (i.e. one clove per day).

- **Kelp tablets** Kelp tablets will help control your metabolic rate and maintain a constant detox state. Ask at your local healthfood shop for a good-quality supplement and follow the daily dosage instructions on the box.

- **Honey** Try to buy a pot from someone who stocks good-quality, home-made honey. The less refined the honey, the better.

- **Fresh lemons** Three to start.

- **Sprouted beans** From your healthfood shop or buy a sprouter and 'do your own'. You can also sprout your own beans on blotting paper or any absorbent paper. Simply dampen the paper, sprinkle on the seeds and leave in a light, sunny place. Make sure the paper doesn't dry out and the beans will sprout in a few days. Mung beans, chickpeas and alfalfa are all good. (If you cannot find these, replace them with a daily supplement of alfalfa pills.)

- **A hot spice of your choice** One or more hot spices, e.g. chilli, cayenne, lemongrass, ginger (raw is best but powdered will do).

- **Water** Filtered or bottled, tap if necessary. Flat is preferable to fizzy – save the fizzy for evenings out! You will need enough for 1.5 litres (3 pints) a day for the first three days.

You can gather these items together in preparation for Day 1 of your Ultimate Detox, but most of the foodstuffs should be bought as and when you would normally do your shopping. The fresher the foods, the more nutrients you will get.

> **Fresh, crisp vegetables will leave you feeling fresh and crisp yourself. Old, limp vegetables . . . need I say more!**

THE COSTS OF THE PROGRAMME

If you do not have some or all of the 'essential items', try to borrow them, as this will keep costs down. If you buy any of these items it will not be a wasted purchase as you will probably continue to use them long after the programme is over. The total cost of steamer, plastic containers and skin brushes or flannels should be less than a good facial – which you will not need as the detox will leave your skin radiant and pure.

Stocking up on the essential foods may mean spending up front at first. But you will recoup the money during the programme, as your fresh foods will cost less than the processed foods that you normally buy.

PROGRAMME SUMMARY

To begin with, here's an at-a-glance summary of the Ultimate Detox programme. The whys and wherefores are all explained later, as you work through the programme in detail. There's a reason for everything on the Ultimate Detox so make sure you do everything on the list and don't eat or drink anything that's not on the food lists in the User's Manual (see pp. 160–4).

THE FOOD PROGRAMME

- Drink a cup of hot water and lemon juice first thing every morning.
- Drink at least 1.5 litres (3 pints) of water during the day
- Take two liver boosters as described on pp. 20–1.
- Take two kidney boosters as described on p. 21.
- Take kelp supplements every day, as directed on the bottle/packet. Do not exceed the recommended maintenance dosage.
- Eat a minimum of three meals and a maximum of five meals every day from the food lists (see User's Manual, pp. 160–4).

- Have at least one portion of short-grain brown rice every day.
- Have at least three portions of vegetables – one should be raw.
- Have at least three portions of raw/fresh or dried fruit.
- Have at least three portions of salad.
- Have at least one portion of non-dairy yoghurt, cheese or milk every day. (Non-dairy means goat's or sheep's products – milk, cheese or yoghurt; rice products – rice milk; or soya products – soya milk.)
- Have two portions of either oily fish, pulses, nuts, olive or any nut or seed oil every day.

THE MIND PROGRAMME

- Say five affirmations every day.
- Treat yourself to something every day.
- Phone a friend every day for a 5-minute chat – time it!
- Give something to someone every day.
- Find something to make you smile or laugh every day.
- Don't make any judgements during the 30 days.
- Take at least four days off.
- Do some gardening every other day.
- Learn something new every week.

THE BODY PROGRAMME

- Have a cold shower or a cold paddle every morning.
- Dry brush your skin every morning.

- Take 30 minutes exercise every day.
- Have 10 minutes relaxation every day.
- Have 5 minutes of quality breathing every day.
- Exfoliate every three days.
- Have an Epsom salts bath every five days.
- Have a professional body treatment every two weeks.

THE FOOD PROGRAMME

In order to get a healthy spread of nutrients you must choose items from all the food lists every day. Missing out on a food category may mean that you begin to feel lethargic as something is missing from your daily requirements. You do not need to have everything for every meal but a sensible combination might be: fruit for breakfast, fish and salad for lunch, roast vegetables and rice for supper, nuts for a mid-morning snack and goat's cheese and rice cakes for dessert. Try to vary this as much as possible but make sure you eat it all! It is important to include raw foods as well as lightly cooked foods. Raw foods provide bulk and roughage which will increase your body's ability to detox.

Drink a cup of hot water and lemon juice first thing every morning

The biggest organ of detox is the liver. Starting the day with a squeeze of fresh lemon juice in a cup of hot water will not only refresh and revitalise you but will also cleanse your palate and help to flush out your liver. Fill the kettle with cold water – bottled or tap. Make sure the water has come to the boil. Then allow to cool a little before adding the lemon juice. The lemon is alkaline-forming, which will help to balance the pH in your system during detox. Drinking this mixture every morning will also help you meet your new daily water intake target and prevent you reaching for the usual tea or coffee.

Drink at least 1.5 litres (3 pints) of water during the day

Our bodies are around 75 per cent water and our brains about 85 per cent water, and we need to keep that level stable. We can go without food for many days but just one or two days without any liquid will result in dehydration and death. We lose water throughout the day, through our skin, our breath, and our kidneys. Water regulates the temperature of our bodies, it keeps our skin moisturised from within, it helps food move through the gut, it flushes out toxic materials, it prevents kidney stones and helps the body avoid urinary infections such as cystitis. Water replenishes, cleanses, rejuvenates and restores and is probably the most important single item in the Ultimate Detox programme. Do you need any more reasons to take the next sip?

In hot weather or during exercise you lose more water than normal so you should increase this amount to cover the deficit. If you detox in the summer or do more exercise, you may require even more. At first this may feel like too much and you will spend a lot of time going to the bathroom! But after a few days your body will become used to the amount and will start to make you thirsty for more. You must be sure to spread this water over the whole day. Drinking it all in one go will put pressure on your internal organs and is not healthy. Reduce the amount you drink leading up to bedtime, as this will prevent you having to get up during the night.

Take two liver boosters as described

The liver is the most important detox organ and as such should be treated with tender loving care during the Ultimate Detox programme. There are many ways to do this but you may find that some are more acceptable than others for your own personal tastes. Each one of the foods below will serve to cleanse and act as a tonic for the liver. If you want to include all of these in your programme that's fine but you must take at least two each day. You can vary the ones you take but make sure you have at least two:

- Eat a medium bunch of red grapes.
- Eat a fresh garlic clove (in your food, not on its own). Or take an odourless garlic tablet every day – a high dose tablet is best.
- Drink a medium glass of either pure carrot or pure beetroot juice (or mix the two). You can make the juice yourself (if you have a juicer) or buy fresh juices from healthfood shops.
- Drink two cups of fennel or dandelion tea.

Take two kidney boosters as described

The other major detox organ is the kidneys. The kidneys balance the body's fluid levels, acidity and alkalinity. Each of the following will boost your kidneys and help the overall programme. Again, you may vary your choice but you must have two per day:

- Have a teaspoon of fresh honey in a cup of hot water. Sip it slowly.
- Drink a medium glass of freshly squeezed cranberry juice (you may wish to add some honey to sweeten) or take a cranberry tablet supplement. NB: Fresh cranberries are generally only available in the winter months, so you may find it easier to take the supplement the rest of the year.
- Eat a large handful of fresh blackcurrants or drink a glass of fresh blackcurrant juice.
- Eat a handful of dried apricots.

Take kelp supplements every day

As explained before, kelp is good for speeding up your metabolic rate and will also help maintain a continuous process of detoxification. Tablets should usually be taken with meals, but follow the instructions provided with your chosen brand. Do not exceed the recommended dosage. If there is a choice, take the maintenance level.

Eat at least three meals every day

During the programme you must eat a minimum of three meals and a maximum of five meals every day from the food lists. It is all too easy to skip a meal due to lack of time or the unavailability of a particular food. But skipping meals will lead to much lower dips in energy and much higher surges that last just a few moments. Eating five or six smaller meals throughout the day is much better for our bodies. Over the next 30 days you should never go longer than four hours without a small meal. Leaving yourself hungry or your stomach empty for long periods will result in your body being exposed to digestive acids. If your hunger becomes too strong you are more likely to crave fatty or sugary foods – none of which are in the food lists (see User's Manual, p. 160–3).

Ideally, you should have breakfast before 9 a.m., lunch before 2 p.m. and your evening meal before 7 p.m. This gives your body sufficient time to digest and absorb the food before your next meal. It also allows your body to process all foods each day before the following day starts. (In a healthy body, foods should normally take less than 24 hours to go from eating to defecation but most people take more than twice that length of time.)

You must have at least one portion of short-grain brown rice every day

Rice is one of the most absorbent carbohydrates we have in our diet. It also seems to avoid the problems of allergic reactions and intolerances that many wheat-based carbohydrates cause. Brown rice promotes good bowel health and keeps blood sugar levels balanced (bread and potatoes give a much sharper rise in blood sugar, resulting in an inevitable drop). Its absorbency means that it can act as a 'plunger' for our lower intestines, and the shorter-grain varieties seem to scour and clean the intestine more thoroughly. Imagine your household pipes after 20 years of use – it is likely that they have either corroded or you have had to call in a plumber to sort out all the minor and major blockages. Brown rice acts like a sponge that travels through your gut, collecting all the silt and waste on the way and then flushing it out. As you are detoxing, each time waste is removed it is not replaced. This means that each time you eat absorbent rice it will break away a little more of the waste until your gut is completely cleansed. Short-grain brown rice is the most absorbent and should be used throughout the programme.

Have at least three portions of vegetables (one should be raw), three portions of raw/fresh or dried fruit, and three portions of salad

Fresh and/or raw vegetables, fruit and salads contain many, many essential nutrients for a healthy and balanced diet. Raw fruit and vegetables contain active ingredients that protect against cancer, heart disease, immune deficiency, deteriorating eyesight and brain dysfunction.

Fruit and vegetables contain large amounts of essential vitamins, amino acids and minerals. They have high fibre and high potassium. They contain very little waste and very few calories. Fruit and vegetables are nearly entirely goodness. You should attempt to eat fresh fruit and vegetables when they are really fresh. The longer you store them, the more nutrients are lost. And as soon as you begin to process or cook them, the goodness starts to disappear. Raw food equals raw energy, it cleans the gut more efficiently and contains high levels of dietary fibre. Try to eat as much as possible of your fruit and vegetable quota in its raw state. Or at least make sure that a high percentage is raw (e.g. raw salad with lightly steamed vegetables). Raw vegetables can also be mixed with cooked vegetables – why not try grated carrot and beetroot over a bowl of grilled vegetables?

Have at least one portion of non-dairy yoghurt, cheese or milk every day

Goat's and sheep's milk products are more easily digested than those made from cow's milk. The fermentation process used in their manufacture means that non-dairy products are easier on the digestive system and, in some cases, can actually stimulate digestion. Many people who have developed an allergy or intolerance to dairy products find they have no reaction to products based on either sheep's or goat's milk. And their nutritional values are virtually identical.

Have two portions of either oily fish, pulses, nuts, olive or seed oil every day

Fish contains essential nutrients, and oily fish has the added benefit of the omega 3 fatty acids. Eating oily fish can lower blood pressure, reduce the risk of heart disease, help protect bones, joints and skin, and is said to protect against some cancers.

Whenever possible you should eat fresh fish. If no fresh is available, or you are using tinned fish for convenience, then the best varieties are those tinned in olive or vegetable oil. Some fish is tinned in spring water but check that no salt has been added. If this is the case, make sure the fish is drained completely and rinsed before eating. Fish in brine is too salty and should not be used on any detox programme. Smoked fish is acceptable but should be naturally smoked and not dyed or coloured.

Fresh fish is always best and will contain the most nutrients.

Naturally smoked and undyed fish can be found both in your supermarket and at the fishmongers. If you cannot find any in stock then you can normally place an order and they can buy it at market especially. They do their shopping more frequently – and earlier! – than we do, and are generally happy to oblige.

Nuts are extremely high in nutrients. Yes, they are high in calories but they are also high in essential unsaturated fatty acids and provide a rich source of potassium and fibre. Nuts should be eaten raw, unsalted and fresh.

Seeds are also high in nutrients, and, once they are freshly sprouted, the nutrient content becomes even higher. Sprouted seeds are easier to digest as they are already partially digested. Seeds and sprouts add flavour and colour to our foods but their vitamin and nutrient content is of ultimate importance.

It's essential to include some fats in your diet but not all fats are good for you. Fats that come in oil form are the best, polyunsaturated. Seed or nut oils should make up part of your everyday diet in order to increase your health substantially. Try using sesame oil, sunflower oil and different nut oils in your salad dressing.

ENTERTAINING

Having friends over for a meal is easy on the Ultimate Detox programme. Fish, olives and herbs are included and vegetables are on the list so you could serve them grilled fish with a herb and olive crust on a bed of chargrilled vegetables drizzled with olive oil. There are many other stunning and delicious combinations that your guests will find hard to believe are part of a detox programme!

PORTION SIZE

The Ultimate Detox programme is very specifically named. It is a *programme* and not a diet. A portion is the same as a heaped tablespoon. Each meal will include a combination of at least 3 portions of either rice, vegetables or miscellaneous foods. Each meal should be a plateful or bowlful. If at any stage you get hungry, then you must eat something, especially in the first half of the programme as your body adjusts. You will probably think that you are eating more than you should – this is quite normal and correct.

Vegetables, fruit and rice provide great sources of carbohydrate and fibre, whilst fish, oil and nuts are good sources of protein and fats. You must make sure that at least two portions of foods such as olive oil, cashew nuts and oily fish are included every day, otherwise your programme will lack the necessary balance. You are not eating any of your normal fats so adding these oily foods is crucial. If you just eat vegetables, rice and fruit you will become tired and your detox process will slow down to a standstill!

The Ultimate Detox programme is not calorie counted but calories are a good way of demonstrating how much you need to eat. Calories are the method we use to measure energy in our food. The average female should eat around 1,600 calories per day and never go below 1,000 calories even when dieting. If the calorie intake is reduced below 1,000 calories we are not providing sufficient energy for our bodies to operate and we go into starvation mode – our bodies store fat for times when they need it, our metabolism slows down, and we become weak and lethargic. It is imperative that you do not let your intake go below the recommended 1,200 calories per day. The Ultimate Detox will only work if you keep all your organs and systems functioning healthily.

COOKING TECHNIQUES

Try to cook your food as little as possible. The less heat the food is subjected to, the more nutrients will remain. Obviously all fish dishes need to be cooked thoroughly but vegetables should always be eaten slightly crisp or al dente. Techniques such as lightly steaming, parboiling, microwaving, stir-frying or flash-frying and grilling are far preferable to boiling or slow cooking as these will reduce both flavour and nutrients.

THE MIND PROGRAMME

Now that you know what you can eat, it is time to look at how you should be thinking, before, during and after your Ultimate Detox.

A healthy body is best combined with a healthy mind. Whilst there are many serious illnesses that cannot be cured through detox, there are also many conditions that can be helped. Taking care of yourself is not a luxury, it is a necessity. Taking care of yourself, your self-esteem and your positive state of mind can only help to promote all-round balanced well-being. The Ultimate Detox programme therefore contains some great tools to get you to look at yourself and your life and to promote positive thinking. Follow these steps every day and see how easy it is to slip into new habits.

Say five affirmations every day

We learn by hearing information and then using it or thinking about it. Well, it's time to learn about yourself, to understand yourself and to make yourself feel good enough for just about anything.

Every morning you should say at least five affirmations. (The User's Manual explains how to decide on your affirmations, see pp. 165–6.) You can say more throughout the day as and when they become useful or necessary or even just as a treat. If you say them in the morning – perhaps as you finish cleaning your teeth – you set the tone for the rest of the day.

Looking at your reflection and thinking, 'I have an awful day ahead of me and I don't know how to get through it', will almost certainly make you even more convinced that it really was not worth getting out of bed. Saying, 'Today will be a great challenge, I am up to it, it will be a breeze, I will be brilliant', is clearly going to get you a lot further.

During the day, as you are experiencing the new challenges, you can say more affirmations: 'You see, you are brilliant, today is going really well, your performance is stunning, just look at how fab you are.'

Each day will have different affirmations and even if things seem really difficult it is still worth squeezing out an affirmation between gritted teeth. It will always work even if your affirmation is 'It cannot get worse than this, I am on the way up, well done.' Repeat this five times and you will really believe it. Affirmations *do* work – they are a great way to boost your mood.

Treat yourself to something every day

This does not mean that you should go out and buy yourself something every day. That is wasted money and not a real treat, as it is meant here. Treating yourself every day means doing little things that have big effects. For instance, you could:

- Allow yourself a lie-in for 30 minutes. (This is easier to time at weekends.)
- Have a long bath in the evening with some wonderful essential oils (see the User's Manual, pp. 178–9). Banish all those muscular aches and stresses.
- Walk around the garden with a cup of tea to see what is growing.
- Read a book for a change.
- Read a magazine that has nothing to do with work.
- Lie down on the sofa with slices of cucumber on your eyes and hand cream on your hands for 15 minutes.
- Go to bed early without having finished the ironing.

Most things that make a huge difference in just a few moments are really very easy to arrange. Just decide what would feel good and do it. A little treat every day is a lot more satisfying than saving up a couple of hours that you never get to use.

Phone a friend every day for a 5-minute chat – time it!

Phone a friend or write them a letter or drop them a card. It should take 5 minutes of your time, just to say hello and catch up on the latest news. If your friend is too far away then write a card or letter or send them something to let them know they were in your thoughts. When you get a little note or answer a call from an old friend you almost certainly smile or have a laugh – it's worth a million and costs almost nothing.

Give something to someone every day

Again, this doesn't have to mean something that costs money. It can be a thought, advice, time, a recipe, an article that they may find interesting, some hand-me-downs for the kids, an article of clothing you no longer wear, a bag of bric-a-brac for the charity shop, permission to take time off work, a thank you for a job well done, a thank you for lunch/supper/an evening together, a listening ear or a friendly postcard. Giving actually makes everyone feel good. If you give with a genuine desire to give then it will be accepted. If you give with a hidden agenda, or expect to receive something in return, then it doesn't work. If in doubt – give a big hug. It works wonders all round.

Find something to make you smile or laugh every day

Laughter has always been the best medicine. Finding something to make you smile or laugh every day will keep your levels of stress down and your health up. Smiling and laughing is a great relaxant. Finding something to make you giggle uncontrollably would be perfect but that isn't always possible. If you know a piece of a film that makes you laugh, or watching your kittens play together gives you a smile, or spending 10 minutes quality time painting, or just playing with your children or a friend's children, then do it.

It's far too easy to take life too seriously. And when you lose your sense of perspective you can forget how to have a good time all too quickly.

Smiling and laughing expands your lungs and uses muscles in your face that keep you looking toned and younger. You see, not only is it good fun but it makes you look and feel great. Find something amusing daily and see how every day can be fun and how much younger you will look and feel.

Don't make any judgements during the 30 days

Many of us spend the whole day making tiny judgements: they're driving too fast, that lipstick doesn't match, he's really annoying, she's in a bad mood, they didn't say thank you, she's really successful, he has no worries, it's all right for them, etc, etc. We make sweeping judgements about almost everything. But if we stopped trying to impose our belief systems on everyone life would be a lot smoother and more relaxed.

One good way of getting rid of bad thoughts or avoiding bad energy or judgement is to place both hands together in front of you, as if beginning a clap, and then swipe the right hand up and off the left hand and away from your body. This signifies that you are 'letting go' of any negativity and stops you making a judgement. For example, if you are in a queue and the person in front has irritated you, simply place your hands together, swipe the right off the left and let that thought go. If you find yourself gossiping or passing comment on someone, again just swipe hands and let it go. If someone asks you what you think about something that is really none of your business, just say it's not for you to judge and go on to another subject.

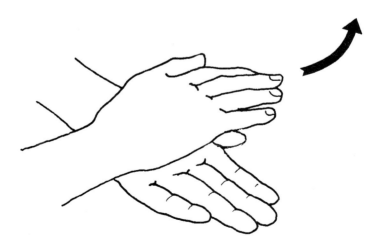

Judging means having to have an opinion on nearly everything but passing no judgement on subjects you don't know anything about frees your mind to concentrate on more important things: How are you feeling? What do you want to do now? What is best for you? . . .

Take at least four days off

These do not need to be together but you must have at least four days to yourself during your month-long programme. Taking time off is difficult to organise. Holidays need to fit in with friends, family, work colleagues and many more. Taking time off when you are supposed to be off (weekends, evenings, early mornings) can be even more difficult! We have developed a culture that says we must be doing something absolutely every moment of the day. We get into work early and stay late to prove we are committed, we join a gym so that we can go before or after work, we travel to see friends most weekends or we fit in a meeting on the way to another meeting.

The Ultimate Detox will rid you of the need to force activities into every spare waking moment and spend some time just 'being'. During this 30-day programme, there must be at least four days where you wake up with *nothing* planned. On these days you can just go with the flow, wake up and take time to think about what you would *like* to do. Even if it turns out that you would *like to do nothing* that's fine. Pretend you are on holiday. Wait to see what the weather suggests, what your mood suggests, whether you want to get dressed . . . Just wait and see how you feel and then go with it and see where you get to. Chill out, relax, lie back, breathe deeply and just be.

Do some gardening every other day

Gardening really means getting on with Mother Earth or Mother Nature, or alternatively getting on with the elements. No matter how much we try to control our environment, it only takes a split second of extreme natural conditions for us to be reminded of just how vulnerable we are to the elements. Unfortunately we only tend to notice Mother Nature's strength when things go wrong. Documentaries about flash floods, avalanches, hurricanes, droughts, famines, mud slides or even sunburn bring home the danger of the elements. But we forget about all those other documentaries on wildlife, rare and beautiful animals, stunning countryside and mountain views. All these things came from the earth or the elements and all these things have immense power to energise and feed us:

- Food comes from the earth in the form of fruit and vegetables.
- Meat comes from the earth in the form of grazing cattle, sheep, hens, etc.
- Fish comes from fresh water or sea water.
- Housing comes from the earth – bricks are made from clay, wood comes from trees.
- Clothing comes from the earth in the form of cotton plants, silk worms, wool from sheep or leather from cows.
- Tools come from the earth in the form of metals from the ground.
- Fuel and heat come from the earth in the form of natural oil, coal, and wood for burning.
- Heat comes from the sun, either directly or via solar power.
- Water comes from the sky, directly or from natural springs that store rain water.

You get the picture. No matter how much we think we supply our own needs, nearly everything we need for our survival comes from the earth, sky or ocean.

We gladly take from the earth without replacing what we have taken. For the duration of the Ultimate Detox programme, and hopefully from this moment forward, you should gain a real understanding of just how important it is to give back.

Gardening gets us out in the air, under the sky, on the earth, or – if we are actually planting or weeding – 'in' the earth. Planting means putting something back into the earth, even if we are planting vegetables to pick later. Weeding or digging means we are helping the earth to be healthy and produce. Just looking at the plants or flowers and taking time to smell them means that we are appreciating the elements and Mother Earth.

Native Americans always sprinkle tobacco – a product of the earth – before taking anything natural, as a gift of thanks. If they have no tobacco then they use coins (metal also comes from the earth). We, in our turn, can pick up litter or plant something or even sprinkle tobacco ourselves to add nutrients to the earth. But the simplest way to say thank you is to do some gardening: tidy up, remove the weeds, water the plants and dig the soil. This uses all the elements, puts back what is lost, relaxes and de-stresses and – you never know – the results might just give you some pleasure as well.

Not having a garden is no excuse. You can still have plants in pots or herbs on a window ledge. These are all ways of getting back to nature and developing a real appreciation of the important things in life.

Learn something new every week

Learning something new uses your mind and your imagination. It cranks up the old grey matter and makes you realise just how long ago it was that you last challenged your head in a positive way.

Learning new things can also save you a lot of effort: not having to look up that phone number every time you call, not having to annoy friends when you call for the second time to ask for a friend's new address, being able to watch a programme you really wanted to because the video can now be programmed without hassle, knowing you will never miss a birthday again or spell that word incorrectly . . .

As you prepare for the Ultimate Detox programme, make a note of four things that would be really good to learn how to do or to remember. Then, during the programme, you can set about completing the tasks. Let your partner/friend/children know what you have planned to do and have them test you at the end of the 30 days.

Well done – what was that about old dogs and new tricks?

THE BODY PROGRAMME

The Ultimate Detox programme is all you will ever need to keep your body in the best possible condition from within. The nutrients from the foods, the internal cleansing actions of the rice, lemon water, fluids, etc, the cleansing of the eliminatory organs, the supplements and 'everyday foods' will all provide a full internal cleanse. However, you also need to look after the outside. There is much more you can do to enhance the vitality of your body and mind through a daily and weekly body care routine.

Have a cold shower or a cold paddle every morning

An invigorating swim in a cool pool, sea or lake every morning would be an 'ideal scenario'. The cold water would increase your circulation, tone muscles and skin and give the lymph a jump start. But if you needed to include a long cool swim every day on the detox programme, alongside all your other new activities, you would soon find yourself spending more time detoxing and less time living your life! Here's an alternative that takes 2 minutes and offers all the benefits of the swim without having to leave your own home – *a cold shower!*

This may sound mad. But if you have ever taken a shower or bath somewhere where there was no hot water you will probably remember that it was a most invigorating experience that actually left you feeling considerably warmer than if you had taken a normal hot shower or bath. Indeed it is more effective in hot weather to take a shower that is luke-warm or blood temperature rather than a cold shower. This is because a cold shower increases your circulation and warms you up instead of cooling you down.

When bathing or showering in the mornings, simply turn the shower to cold just before you are ready to finish and let the icy cold water run over your entire body for just 1 minute. Alternatively, when you have finished your bath you can turn on the cold tap as the bath water is draining away, cup your hands under the water and splash it all over your body.

If you happen to live by the sea then any chance you get you should take off your shoes and paddle (but only for a maximum of 2 minutes – we don't want any reports of frostbite!).

Dry brush your skin every morning

This once unheard-of process now appears in every health and beauty magazine – and quite right too! Sloughing away dead skin cells helps remove any barriers to your skin 'breathing' efficiently. It clears the pores, and improves the appearance of the skin. (Dead skin is dull and does not reflect light well, whereas healthy skin glows in normal light conditions.)

Brushing also improves blood and lymph circulation. The brushing action does this by stimulating muscle contraction to help the lymph and blood flow. The improved lymph flow leads to more efficient excretion of waste materials in the cells and interstitial fluid. And this encourages more efficient cell production and renewal.

Increasing the flow of interstitial fluid also causes the excess fluids to drain and clear from the often troublesome hip and thigh areas. Water retention (or oedema) can thus be prevented with more efficient fluid and lymph flow.

In addition, brushing stimulates the production of sebum which in turn helps to improve the texture and tone of the skin. For clear, instructions on how to carry out effective dry skin brushing, see the User's Manual (pp. 167–8).

The whole process should only take 3 or 4 minutes. Your skin will tingle and you should feel quite warm, as you will have stimulated and increased your circulation. You will soon notice quite a difference in your skin. It will feel smoother, with a softer texture and the dry patches will all have disappeared. Just spend a little time each day and you will be pleasantly surprised.

Take 30 minutes exercise every day

Exercise is one of the best ways to enhance the Ultimate Detox programme. It costs nothing, it can be done at any time of the day or night (even whilst you are doing everyday chores) and it has many, many benefits. The Fitness Association in the UK has issued a list of good reasons to take exercise. The highlighted reasons below are those that are particularly relevant to this detox programme:

- Promotes gains in stamina
- Improves neuro muscular co-ordination
- Relieves symptoms of menopause
- Increases the body's ability to fight off infection
- May help prevent heart disease
- Reduces risk of glaucoma
- Helps prevent osteoporosis
- Reduces the risk of breast cancer
- Decreases the risk of colon cancer
- Lessens arthritic pain
- Lowers blood pressure
- Controls cholesterol
- Reduces the risk of obesity
- Burns fat
- Burns calories
- Speeds up metabolism
- Relieves constipation
- Alleviates PMT
- Helps prevent endometriosis
- Helps stop smoking

- Reduces alcohol consumption
- Relieves depression
- Releases anxiety
- Reduces stress
- Improves sexual performance
- Enhances self-esteem
- Heightens sense of well-being
- Improves mental sharpness
- Increases IQ
- Improves concentration
- Enhances creativity
- Improves outlook
- Decreases job absenteeism
- Reduces medical costs
- Increases productivity
- Increases job satisfaction
- Improves flexibility
- Preserves muscle
- Improves circulation
- Preserves functional capacity
- Increases mobility
- Improves memory
- Improves reaction time
- Shortens rehabilitation after illness or injury
- Increases range of motion
- Improves cardiovascular fitness
- Promotes a healthy back
- Deepens sleep
- Increases energy
- Lengthens life

Now that you have so many good reasons to take exercise, you should do at least 30 minutes every day during your Ultimate Detox programme. Not only will this help to keep you fit and toned but it will also ensure that your metabolic rate does not decrease or your circulation become sluggish.

Little and often is also much better than spending two hours every two weeks. One long session is more likely to tire you out, you will not build up any benefit from your exercise as it happens too infrequently, and it will be discouraging and you are very likely to give up. If you exercise for 30 minutes every day, it doesn't interfere with your day too much, it's over before you get bored and you will notice the benefits after just a few days. You are also more likely to get inspired. Soon 30 minutes will become

40 minutes, until you build up to a level of exercise that suits you and your lifestyle.

Exercise tips

Getting started is the hardest part. But if you think about your daily routine you may find that you can slip in the exercise without even noticing. For example:

- If you normally start the day by going downstairs to get the post or to make breakfast, try going up and down the stairs three times before you boil the kettle.

- If you normally drive to school to pick up the children, walk.

- You could jog whilst vacuuming or stretch for 5 minutes whilst dusting.

- If you are going to sit in a meeting for several hours go to the meeting room via the longest route and run up and down the stairs several times before sitting down.

- In the evening, whilst watching television, you can lift and lower your legs, or tense and relax your stomach muscles several times.

- When everyone is out of the house, turn the music up and dance for 30 minutes – this feels great and it's good exercise as well!

- Instead of going out to a bar, go to a nightclub and dance.

- Go rollerblading rather than walking on Sunday.

- Don't watch the kids in the pool, get in there with them.

- Sit in the bath and do stretches from side to side or scissor your legs together and apart using the water as weights – be careful not to splash too much!

Of course the more traditional methods of exercise are still very valuable – joining a gym, going to exercise classes, playing sport, jogging, etc, but if you have tried all these and not found your natural form of exercise, don't be discouraged. Set yourself a challenge to find the most unusual form of exercise you can, and do it for 30 minutes each day.

If you are the type of person who likes to watch sequences then get a video exercise tape of someone you like and admire. Work with this, gradually building up the amount of time you spend, until you can do the whole tape without blinking.

If you are the type of person who likes to follow a sequence in a book then please refer to the User's Manual (pp. 168–70) which will take you through an elementary routine that you can do yourself.

All the exercises, except the jogging, should be slow and deliberate. And you should use your body weight as resistance, to increase the effectiveness of the exercises. You can build up the repetitions as soon as you become comfortable with the programme. Do them for as long as you wish, as long as you do at least 30 minutes every day.

Posture is also an important part of exercise. We are all designed so that our internal organs have sufficient space to operate efficiently. If we change this, by putting on weight, losing weight, sitting with our bodies squashed, or slumping whilst we eat, then our organs need to compensate. This will lead to problems such as: inefficient expansion of the lungs whilst breathing, lack of oxygen in the body, incorrect absorption of vital vitamins and minerals, indigestion, poor circulation and headaches. More obvious physical effects occur as well, including slouching shoulders, weak stomach muscles and a concave chest. Exercise will keep the body and muscles in a condition that will prevent any of these effects from occurring or will correct any that have already set in.

Whatever form of exercise you choose you should treat it as something that you deserve, which enhances your detox programme. It's easy to think of exercise as hard work and a chore, something that both your mind and body have to endure, when actually both your body and mind love exercise and need it to function efficiently.

Have 10 minutes relaxation every day

If you are fit and healthy and 'detoxed' then relaxation can be a continual state. This is not to say that you will just laze around, never doing anything. It actually means that you will do things in a way that does not harm your body or put you under any unnecessary stress. For example, you can be presenting to 500 delegates at a conference but still remain relaxed, or you can stand in a queue at the supermarket with four impatient children and still remain relaxed – if you just use some simple techniques.

Once you have combined exercise and correct breathing, it is very easy to keep yourself feeling in control, calm, confident and relaxed.

We have discussed breathing and how important that is to staying relaxed. We have also discussed visualisation and affirmations (see p. 27) and how these can give you confidence and help you achieve your goals. If you truly believe that you will get everything you want in life, and you are 'centred and grounded' with regular deep breathing, then you will achieve true relaxation. Of course there are bound to be a few hurdles and hiccups along the way but if the future holds all you desire then relaxation is natural.

A simple relaxation exercise is featured in the User's Manual (see pp. 170–2). Follow it every day and feel the flow of calm. The more you actively practise these relaxation techniques, the easier they become. As with the breathing exercises, you will soon be able to take yourself into deep relaxation at any time, day or night. Memorise the sequence, or say it into a tape very slowly and play it to yourself as you are relaxing.

Have 5 minutes of quality breathing every day

Everyone knows how important oxygen, fresh air and good breathing are for our survival. But if you ask anyone exactly how to breathe correctly, or what effects good breathing has, they will probably struggle to give you an answer.

The fact is that even a momentary lack of the correct levels of oxygen in the body will result in serious damage and eventually death. Yet many of us continue to underuse the capacity of our lungs and deprive our bodies of all the benefits that correct breathing will bring. From early childhood we are told to 'stand up straight, stomachs in', and when we are told to take a deep breath we automatically inhale and raise our chest. Yet, by restricting movement of the stomach and abdomen, we are limiting the area the lungs can expand into. And so we develop the habit of only using a third of our lung capacity each time we inhale.

Balance of mind and body is also affected by breathing. If you are tense and stressed and your breathing is short and shallow, you are less likely to be able to think straight. Your movements become erratic and your balance is thrown.

Correct breathing is easy and more relaxing, and simple breathing exercises can be carried out whenever you feel it necessary.

To breathe correctly you simply relax your stomach muscles, inhale through your nose slowly and take in the air until it feels as if the base of your stomach is full of air. Pause for a moment and then exhale through the mouth. Feeling 'the air in your stomach' shows that you have relaxed your diaphragm muscle, which means your lungs have fully expanded and you have inhaled to full capacity. This will feel strange at first but will soon become the normal way to breathe and you won't need to think about it any more.

Deeper breathing slows the heart rate and the pulse; and the deeper we breathe, the more oxygen we inhale. All these factors lead to improved health.

Exfoliate every three days

Exfoliation has all the benefits of the dry skin brushing technique, but can be included as part of the more relaxing, tranquil or even indulgent times in your Ultimate Detox programme. Exfoliation needs water and some form of home-made or cosmetic exfoliant. It is generally gentler on the skin and it can therefore be used on the face and any delicate areas that might find dry brushing a little too harsh. Exfoliating products are widely available in all price ranges and are usually combined with wonderfully scented creams or gels. However, if you do not wish to buy an exfoliating scrub you can easily make you own. There is a recipe to follow in the User's Manual (see p. 174).

Have an Epsom salts bath every five days

Magnesium is necessary for nearly all the cellular activity in our bodies. Epsom salts are pure magnesium, so bathing in Epsom salts allows the skin to absorb the magnesium. The magnesium will also absorb or 'draw' toxins from the body, so it is likely that you will 'glow' with perspiration for a while after your bath. This will not be quite a sweat – unless you wrap up really warm! – but is more likely to feel like being in a very humid room. It is vital to keep warm, not only to increase the effects of the magnesium but also to prevent you from catching a chill. Epsom salts baths will improve circulation and speed up the elimination of toxins.

An Epsom salts bath can also be extremely relaxing and warming, helping to soothe aching joints and muscles. Taken before bed, it will almost certainly guarantee the deepest night's sleep!

There are instructions on how to make the ideal Epsom salts bath in the User's Manual (see pp. 175–6).

Have a professional body treatment every two weeks

There are many treatments available today that you can get quite readily from your local health club or beauty salon. They can range from facials, manicures and pedicures, through to massage using heated and frozen stones. They can be very clinical, or they can be extremely spiritual. They can work with your physical body, or they can work on your emotions. Whatever your particular needs, there will be one that is perfect for you. You need to take some time to research the treatments; read about them, ask the therapist about them or even go along to a demonstration and then choose the ones that most appeal to you.

Some massage can be very deep and some can be very light. Some treatments can work on an energetic level above the body, and in some treatments the therapist will physically lift and move body parts around. Whatever treatment you decide upon, it is likely to be based on some form of massage and massage is fabulous for any detox programme because it:

- Warms and relaxes the muscles
- Relieves tension
- Reduces stress
- Increases the blood circulation
- Increases lymph flow
- Helps to improve the immune system
- Helps the body eliminate excess fluids
- Helps the body eliminate waste products
- Improves the flow of interstitial fluid, improving the appearance of the skin, especially in areas prone to cellulite
- Lowers blood pressure

- Tones the muscles
- Tones the skin
- Provides a passive work-out for the whole body

MASSAGE TREATMENTS

Massage, alongside aromatherapy, is one of the oldest forms of complementary therapy known. As with aromatherapy, massage can be done in isolation (for example, face massage or foot massage) or in total (a full body massage incorporating every part of the body including stomach and abdomen).

Traditional massage works by increasing the circulation, which in turn helps the efficient flow of lymph. This has a positive effect on the immune system and keeps the body balanced and healthy. During the Ultimate Detox programme any therapy that enhances these functions should be encouraged and enjoyed as much as possible. Muscle conditions involving soreness and tension are all helped with massage, as the increased blood flow and the manipulation will help to stretch and tone. There are many other benefits (e.g. improved skin tone, relaxed mind, lowered heart rate and so on).

Massage is often described as 'Swedish' or 'therapeutic' or 'holistic'. In fact there is not much difference between these as all massage strokes derive from three original 'Swedish' techniques: *effleurage*, *pettrissage* and *tapotement*. *Effleurage* (flat hands pushing flesh from the lower body, up towards the head and back down the body) to warm the muscles and flesh and to increase the circulation prior to deeper work. *Pettrissage* (kneading, wringing and pulling the muscles so that the flesh and muscles are worked against each other or the flesh is pressed against the bone to cause deeper friction) is used to tone the muscles and flesh and to work through any tension or spasm. And *tapotement* involves quick, invigorating strokes, such as *hacking* (where the side of the hand is used to 'chop' the flesh), *cupping* (where cupped hands are placed in rapid succession on the flesh to 'draw' the blood to the surface) or *pummelling* (where the hands are clenched in fist shapes and placed flesh down in rapid succession on the flesh to cause deeper impression on the muscles and increase circulation).

There are many other types of massage, including remedial, sports, Thai, Indian head, etc. All of these are very valuable but for the detox process the traditonal aromatherapy and massage techniques are the best.

During a massage the client will lie on a couch, either naked or in their underwear. They will be covered in towels or a blanket and the room should be warm and calm. All massage strokes should be carried out 'towards the heart' (or 'venous return'), as this helps complete the passage of blood throughout the body and increases the circulation of both blood and lymph.

Initial strokes should be relaxing, warming and smooth and should not cause any pain. There may be some discomfort but there should be no actual pain. Strokes should work in time with your breathing and follow a regular pace. As the treatment progresses and the muscles have been warmed then the strokes can become more rigorous and more intrusive, as the practitioner 'milks' the muscles of any toxins and drains the body of any wastes.

Once an area has been warmed, very deep, specific work can be carried out. This may feel uncomfortable but will help to sort out deep-seated problems or tense muscles.

Whatever the reason for your massage, it should give you an overall feeling of relaxation and well-being. If carried out correctly, you may feel 'worked over' yet invigorated, and not exhausted, in pain or bruised.

During a detox, massage is wonderful. The lighter strokes relax and warm you, the deeper strokes sort out your muscles and increase your circulation to help the internal cleansing process, and the invigorating strokes stimulate and give you a truly vital feeling. Massage is perhaps my favourite choice of professional treatment.

Massage practitioners will use an oil such as the base or carrier oils used in in aromatherapy, or they will use a blend of carrier oils and some basic essential oils.

People often, mistakenly, think that aromatherapy and massage are the same thing. Aromatherapy massage treatments are designed to facilitate the optimum absorption of the essential oils. The treatment warms the flesh, and this increases the circulation so that the body can totally absorb the oils. It is the oils that trigger effects within the body and not the physical treatment itself. Massage treatments are designed to improve the circulation, lymph flow and immune system entirely through the physical use of different speed, length and pressure of strokes. You will feel much more 'worked' after a massage treatment than you should after an aromatherapy treatment. Each of these techniques is valuable in its own right, and you should be aware of the differences in order to decide on the best approach for you.

AROMATHERAPY TREATMENTS

> **Important Note**
>
> Please note that essential oils should never be used if you believe you are pregnant or if you are trying to become pregnant, unless prescribed by a trained aromatherapist. Essential oils should never be taken internally.

Aromatherapy uses plant-extracted essential oils. Many people wrongly believe that it is simply nice-smelling massage. In fact, aromatherapy is much, much more than this. It can become an essential part of your everyday life and, more specifically, an essential part of any detoxification programme. There is a lengthier description in the User's Manual (see pp. 176–8) of the history of essential oils and how to use them safely and effectively. There are also details of how aromatherapy oils have been used traditionally in massage, and information on bathing, burners, ready-made blends and their uses, and how to choose good quality essential oils. There is also a brief description of some useful oils to have around the home and their therapeutic qualities.

Essential oils are absorbed into our bodies via the skin or the olfactory system (inhalation). The skin is a semi-permeable membrane and the transfer of the essential oil molecules through the skin into the bloodstream means that the effects can begin as soon as the oils are applied to the skin. They will continue as long as the oils are on the surface of the flesh. Once in the bloodstream, the molecules will travel to the brain and trigger the necessary functions relevant to the specific oil used. (Initial doubt as to whether substances can be absorbed through the skin has been eliminated by the introduction of 'patches' for many conditions by the medical industry.)

When we inhale the essential oil fragrance the molecules travel inside the nostrils and reach the brain through the thin membranes in the nasal passages and the olfactory system. Inhaling the oils is the quickest way to benefit from them.

During an aromatherapy massage treatment the client is required to lie on a massage couch, either naked or in their underwear, covered in towels or blankets. The room should be warm and the practitioner should have a calm, relaxing approach. The treatment will usually last about an hour. You may feel drowsy after the session but a glass of water will soon remedy this.

LaStone therapy

LaStone therapy is a relatively new treatment based on extremely old foundations. LaStone therapy is massage using heated basalt stones and frozen marble stones. The treatment was invented by a lady called Mary Hannigan, in Tuçson, Arizona. It combines thermotherapy (use of hot and cold) with spiritual and energy work, and leaves the client feeling balanced, grounded, renewed and positive.

The treatment itself is similar to massage and aromatherapy. You lie on a couch, covered in towels, and the practitioner uses long and short massage strokes to work over the body. However, in this case, the therapist has a hot or cold stone in their hand throughout the treatment.

Essential oils can be incorporated into the treatment. Alternatively, the therapist will simply use a base oil to help the stones work across the flesh. People who have had the treatment report that it is like being comforted or returning to the womb. The small stones feel like lots of little hot-water bottles being tucked in against the skin, and the cool stones are refreshing and invigorating. It's a treatment that's really worth trying if you get the chance.

COLONIC IRRIGATION

Colonic irrigation has been around since as early as 1500 BC, but still seems to be a relatively new and experimental therapy for most people.

Colonic irrigation is an internal bath that helps to cleanse the colon of accumulated poisons, gases, faecal matter and mucous deposits. The practitioner will gently pump filtered water into the rectum and this will start to soften and flush away any unwanted build-up of toxins and waste.

Colonic irrigation is extremely effective during any detox programme. During the programme you eliminate all toxins from your diet. There will still be a build-up of toxins within the body from before the programme but foodstuffs such as brown rice, nuts and pulses all help to break this down. Colonic irrigation will speed up this breakdown process and will actively flush out any waste matter.

The colonics practitioner will ask you to lie on a couch or plinth, with your lower body covered with a towel or sheet. Filtered water at a carefully regulated temperature is introduced under gentle gravitational pressure through the rectum and into the colon. The practitioner will use massage to help the water soften and cleanse the colon of faecal matter and waste, which will be flushed away with the waste water. The colon is worked on in stages; each time water is pumped in and flushed out until the whole area is complete. The treatment will last less than an hour and the modesty of the client is observed throughout – practitioners are totally aware of the 'unusual' circumstances that they place their clients in. It is usual for the practitioner to advise on how many further treatments are required and also which supplements are needed to replace natural bowel fibre and flora.

The after-effects of colonic irrigation are similar to those of the entire Ultimate Detox programme: a sense of well-being, lightness, mental clarity, increased energy, loss of bloated feeling, relief from constipation and clearer, glowing skin.

Colonics may not immediately spring to mind as a complementary therapy – we normally think of massage or aromatherapy – but if you have ever wondered about trying this treatment, now's the time! It's painless, it's different, it makes you feel great and it's detoxifiying.

REFLEXOLOGY

Reflexology is based on the principle that there are reflex points or zones on the feet which relate to points, organs and systems within the body. By working with these zones or points the practitioner can treat areas of illness, imbalance or weakness.

Reflexology has been recorded as far back as Egyptian times and Eunice Ingham documented the practice in the early 1900s. Ingham was a physiotherapist who believed that there were many zones running through and connecting the body. She believed that these could be more easily accessed and worked on in certain parts of the body, i.e. the feet. It was this work that developed into the therapy of reflexology as we know it today.

During a reflexology treatment, the client sits or lies on a couch and the practitioner follows a manipulation sequence around each foot, covering every reflex point or zone. The practitioner will require feedback from the client concerning areas of discomfort or pain during the treatment. The practitioner can then 'work' the relevant area to improve the condition. Reflexology practitioners tend to use powders, such as calendula or talcum, to make the treatment go smoothly. Reflexology is an excellent diagnostic tool, as it can show any problems, even at the early stages, within the body. The practitioner can then work on them before any further, more serious, conditions develop.

During the Ultimate Detox programme your internal systems and organs will probably be working harder or differently from the way they would normally. Reflexology can help the body detox by 'balancing' organs like the kidneys and liver, and enabling the intestines to carry out their cleansing function without causing any unnecessary pressure. Reflexology can also tell you what your body requires or simply what it is going through. If you have reflexology treatments whilst you are detoxing you will find that common 'tender points' are those of the bladder, kidney and digestive systems, all of which are working hard. The practitioner will work on these specific points to bring them to optimum condition for continued cleansing.

Reflexology treatments will also show any potential imbalance and the practitioner can work at a preventative level. If you are super-healthy or your detox has made your body totally balanced, then reflexology treatments are still useful as a precaution and as a time to relax.

There are some basic reflex points that you can work on yourself every day to instill calmness and health:

- The 'great eliminator', located in the fleshy part of your hand between the thumb and forefinger, can be used to expel stress and tension. Using the thumb and forefinger of your left hand, gently squeeze this fleshy area on your right hand. You should apply pressure slowly as it may well be tender, especially if you have a headache or are feeling tense. Hold the pressure and release slowly; repeat until you feel the tension or the headache subside. When you feel ready, swap hands and release tension on the other hand.

- The 'centre point' in the palm of your hand relates to the centre point on your solar plexus (chest area) and the centre point on your foot; obviously the easiest point to reach is your hand. Place your left thumb in the centre of your right palm, supporting the weight of the right hand with the fingers of the left hand. Slowly move the thumb upwards towards the fingers and stop when you meet the underside of the knuckles – just off centre from the palm towards the fingers. Again, apply pressure slowly and hold it until the pressure subsides. Repeat for the other hand and feel the tension melt away.

- The zone points on your face can be worked by placing both thumbs just inside the eye socket, up against the brow bone. Place your elbows on your desk or a table and then lower the weight of your head onto your thumbs. Again this may feel tender, especially if you are trying to eliminate a headache. Hold the pressure and then release.

YOGA

Yoga is the physical version of meditation. You use your body to effect a change on your mind and body instead of simply your breathing. But be warned – yoga is not a simple form of exercise for stretch 'n' tone. Some of the advanced techniques look as if they are completely above and beyond the bounds of human flexibility but they really are quite possible if you build up to them gradually. Having a relaxed mind will enable your body to 'work out' the moves. Attempting them without relaxation is likely to cause injury. After practising yoga for a while, you will find a sense of emotional, physical and mental calm.

Yoga will tone your muscles. It will also tone your internal systems and organs, as some of the positions exert pressure on them or release them and their surrounding areas. It will keep your joints supple and your spine healthy, supportive and strong. Each yoga position has a special purpose. A yoga session will work all aspects of the body and free everything up so that you achieve mental and physical clarity. Breathing into moves and holding them requires concentration and balance. There is nothing quick or sharp about yoga. Actually getting your body into some of the positions safely requires a process of gentle stretches, holding and concentration.

As with meditation, you should always start by attending a class or having lessons with a qualified, experienced yoga teacher. The yoga class will consist of relaxation and warming exercises, followed by a series of positions that may take some time to achieve. Then there will be more relaxation and balancing, before a further position is attempted. You are likely to need lots of blankets, pillows, pads and layers of clothes, as the class goes from still and meditative, through physical, and back to stretching and relaxation. Always check what is required when you register with a class and make sure the teacher knows your level.

Tai Chi

Tai Chi dates back to ancient China – as far as 3000 BC. It is really only now, nearly 5,000 years later, that we Westerners have decided there may be something in it! Tai Chi literally means 'big energy'. It involves becoming aware of our own personal energy and the energy surrounding us and working in harmony with these energies.

Everything has energy, and Tai Chi helps us recognise it for ourselves. Tai Chi is also exercise; through performing some graceful balletic movements we begin to feel the flow of energy, both inner and outer.

As with all Oriental treatments, once you have got to grips with the basics, you can practise Tai Chi safely almost anywhere you wish.

Tai Chi has indeed become famous because so many people go out every day to an open space and practise there. The energy (or Chi) actually changes at around 3–4 a.m. every day and devout practitioners will tell you that dawn exercise is one of the most amazing ways to experience Tai Chi. However, it is perhaps a little more practical to begin in your own home or gym in order to feel comfortable before you start to 'go public'.

Shiatsu

Shiatsu is another Oriental art that involves working with the body to increase health.

The Chinese use acupuncture and acupressure and the Japanese use Shiatsu, which is the use of firm pressure on different points of the body that relate to different energy paths or specific organs. This works in a very similar way to the points and meridians used in acupuncture and reflexology.

Pressure physically applied to particular points, using elbows, knees, fingers and many other parts of the body, will invigorate the client and will clear any blockages in energy, resulting in fitness and balanced flow.

This brief overview should have given you a good idea of some of the treatments that are available. You will find relevant contact numbers and addresses in the User's Manual (see pp. 193–5).

CHECK LIST

Now that you are aware of all aspects of the 30-Day Ultimate Detox, you can go on to actually plan your own programme.

To help you remember to do everything, there is a list below. Make sure that you tick each box as you carry out the instruction and then you can be sure that nothing has been left out:

- ☐ Drink a cup of hot water and lemon juice first thing every morning.
- ☐ Drink at least 1.5 litres (3 pints) of water during the day.
- ☐ Take two Liver Boosters as described on pp. 20–1.
- ☐ Take two Kidney Boosters as described on p. 20.
- ☐ Take kelp supplements every day.
- ☐ Eat a minimum of three meals and a maximum of five meals every day from the food lists (see User's Manual, pp. 160–3).
- ☐ Have at least one portion of short-grain brown rice every day.
- ☐ Have at least three portions of vegetables – one should be raw.
- ☐ Have at least three portions of raw/fresh or dried fruit.
- ☐ Have at least three portions of salad.
- ☐ Have at least one portion of non-dairy yoghurt, cheese or milk every day. (Non-dairy means goat's or sheep's products – milk, cheese or yoghurt; rice products – rice milk; or soya products – soya milk.)
- ☐ Have two portions of either oily fish, pulses, nuts, olive or any nut or seed oil every day.
- ☐ Say five affirmations every day.
- ☐ Treat yourself to something every day.

- [ ] Phone a friend every day for a 5-minute chat — time it!
- [ ] Give something to someone every day.
- [ ] Find something to make you smile or laugh every day.
- [ ] Don't make any judgements during the 30 days.
- [ ] Take at least four days off.
- [ ] Do some gardening every other day.
- [ ] Learn something new every week.
- [ ] Have a cold shower or cold paddle every morning.
- [ ] Dry brush your skin every morning.
- [ ] Take 30 minutes exercise every day.
- [ ] Have 10 minutes relaxation every day.
- [ ] Have 5 minutes of quality breathing every day.
- [ ] Exfoliate every three days.
- [ ] Have an Epsom salts bath every five days.
- [ ] Have a professional body treatment every two weeks.

2 The Quick-Fix Hangover Detox

For those times when you have just too good a time and end up overdoing it, this programme has some handy hints on ways to spend the morning and day after. Advice on supplements, exercise and attitude will help to get you through the over-indulgence and apologise to your body for the abuse. There are also ways to prevent anything like that happening again – the 'never again' solutions.

THE TRUTH ABOUT HANGOVERS

Alcohol in excess is damaging to your body. The hangover is exactly that, the 'hang over' from the night before (or the after-effects of alcoholic drinks on your body). Quite simply, you poison your body and it reacts badly. No surprise there. There have been frequent reports about the nutritional value of alcohol. It's sometimes argued that it can be beneficial in some cases, in regulated amounts. But, whatever the findings, it is

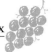

generally agreed that alcohol in excess is damaging, addictive and destructive.

The only way to avoid these effects is not to drink to excess. This Hangover Detox should in no way give the impression that you can drink to excess with no ill-effects from now on. On the contrary, excess drinking is bad for you, your body and your long-term health. And if you think you may have an alcohol addiction problem then please seek professional advice immediately.

What this programme does set out to do is help you through the moments we all have in our lives when we have overdone it and are suffering the consequences. Given that most of us like to have a drink now and then, and most of us, at one time or another, drink more than the recommended amount, there are several ways to make this insult to our bodies less damaging to our internal and external organs.

Hangovers affect people in many different ways but some of the more common side-effects of excessive drinking are: headaches, nausea, dehydration and tiredness. The internal effects are even grimmer. As the organ that processes the alcohol, the liver suffers the most damage. The skin is the largest organ of elimination, so when your body takes in excess toxins your complexion takes the strain. Your stomach becomes very acidic,

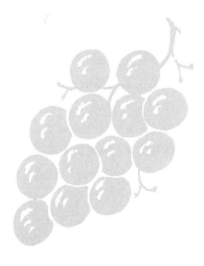

due to the alcohol, and the nausea sets in. Your intestines are sluggish, and you are likely to experience wind and softer stools. Dehydration means your insides are beginning to feel prune-like and very unsavoury.

To make matters worse, the types of foods most of us crave after a big night out are never conducive to repair or recovery: black coffee, greasy breakfast and lots of toast. It all feels very comforting and the principles are very honourable: to wake up (the coffee), absorb the excesses (the toast), and fill a stomach that is churning and empty (the greasy fry-up). But the coffee is a diuretic, which will not only get rid of any fluid your body has left, it will also encourage loss of any water you have drunk to try to recover.

The caffeine will also add to the problems your liver is currently dealing with by forcing it to cleanse and purify before flushing out. The toast will fill your body with starch, carbohydrate and sugars, all of which will increase the acidity of your stomach. The hot dripping butter has no effect on the acidity and is highly calorific – although at least reasonably natural! All this will lull you into a false sense of well-being due to a slight increase in energy levels.

The fry-up is no help either. The transient jump in energy levels leads you to believe that you have turned the corner. But the bacon, eggs and fried bread are all acid-forming. The only saving grace is the mushrooms and grilled tomatoes which are alkaline-forming. Along with all this, you have taken in a heap of calories and toxins to add to your problems. No wonder your liver is starting to protest.

If your body is in tip-top condition then you may find that the occasional over-indulgence like this will simply mean that you feel tired and listless the following day. But if your body has been working hard, if you have been getting by on takeaways and processed foods, if your diet contains little or no fresh fruit and vegetables, if your fluid intake is made up of hourly caffeine injections, then all the symptoms will apply. A thoroughly rotten day or even several days can be expected and the words 'never again' will be muttered from beneath what feels like the head from hell.

BEFORE YOU START DRINKING

If you know there is a possibility that you will over-indulge one day or evening then you should at least prepare your body.

Protecting against dehydration

The main side-effect is dehydration. Drinking at least 1.5 litres (3 pints) of water in the several days leading up to the big night out (you should be drinking this amount every day as a matter of course) will help your body in two main ways. Firstly, it will completely hydrate your body in preparation for the alcohol which will increase the rate of fluid loss. Secondly, it will help your body to cleanse by leaving it fully purged and ready to deal with flushing through the alcohol to come.

Protecting your liver

The liver is the organ of cleansing and detoxification so, over the next days, you need to keep it fully cleansed and ready for the overtime to come. There are many liver tonics and these are described in detail in the 30-Day Ultimate Detox (see pp. 20–1). Include plenty of beetroot, black grapes, fresh garlic and garlic pills (odourless are best). Eat carrots or drink carrot juice – you can combine this with other juices but make sure you include plenty of carrot and/or beetroot. Fennel and dandelion tea should also form part of your diet for the days preceding a big night out.

Protecting your stomach

There are also things you can do to prepare and even 'line' your stomach to help the alcohol pass through without too many problems. Blood sugar levels should be maintained and extremes should be avoided. Eat full meals during the day and don't have your first drink on an empty stomach. Make sure your meals consist of plenty of vegetables, brown rice, salads, fruit, etc.

If there is no healthy food available – often the nibbles are dips or fried food or are high in salt to make you drink more – just make sure you eat something, as drinking on a full stomach is much healthier for your stomach and will probably mean you drink less.

During the evening

You can also take steps throughout the festivities that will help to ensure minimum damage the following day:

- When choosing your drink remember that mixing sugar with alcohol – sweet spirits – will speed up the absorption of the alcohol, making you get drunk quicker. For this reason you should avoid spirits and sweet sugary drinks like alcopops or pre-mixed bottled drinks. Sugary drinks will also make you drink more as the sugar high you get will soon fall and you will reach for another drink just to keep your energy up.

- Keep your hydration levels up by matching every alcoholic drink with the same amount of water. This doesn't mean you have to dilute your drinks but it does mean that every other drink could be water. If you think that drinking water is not possible because the host will pressurise you to have a good time then fake it. A sparkling water with ice and lemon in a spirit glass can look like a gin or vodka and tonic and no one need ever know the difference. Barmen are very good at not giving the game away.

- You can make a long drink out of white wine by creating a spritzer – more fluid, less alcohol.

- Remember how you will feel the next day. Cutting back or stopping when you feel you've had enough is the best answer. Even then there is probably still enough alcohol in your system to have done quite enough damage and some that hasn't even had time to take effect. Stopping when you feel jolly is probably already too late but will at least guarantee a fun evening and a clearer head the next day.

- Drink plenty of fluids before you go to bed. Put some fresh lemon juice in your water – this is alkaline-forming and will decrease the acidity of your stomach.

- Each time you wake in the night to go to the toilet, make sure you replace what you have lost. Have a glass beside the bed and take six mouthfuls before you drift back off to fitful sleep.

- Sweet dreams.

THE FOLLOWING DAY

Today will go slowly and you must listen to your body. It did what you wanted to do yesterday so it is time to treat it gently and do as it asks. Don't try anything strenuous. You have filled your body with poison so give it a chance to get back to full fitness in its own time.

RECOVERY TIPS

- **Drink water upon rising.**

This rehydrates you. Sips are better than overloading with a whole glass in one go. Aim for about 250 ml (½ pint) every half-hour.

- Have hot water, lemon juice and a dash of honey in place of caffeine. Drink as much as you want.

  This reduces the acidity of your stomach and balances your blood sugar levels.

- Make yourself a breakfast of muesli, yoghurt, fresh fruit, nuts and seeds. (No matter how tempted you are to resort to the fry-up, just don't. Eat more museli if you need to nibble but don't go greasy. Just think of the grease, oil and fats all churning up inside, compared to the absorbent oats, nuts and fruits.)

  This balances your stomach acidity and blood sugar, and provides good solid nutritious energy with no sugar slump afterwards.

- Drink peppermint tea and plenty of water throughout the day.

  This rehydrates you some more and settles your digestion.

- Drink a little fizzy water.

  Carbonated water helps to re-oxygenate your blood.

- Eat plenty of fresh vegetables, fruits, salads, brown rice, non-dairy cheeses and yoghurts, grilled fish, seeds, nuts and pulses.

  These foods will keep your energy levels steady.

Take it easy

Relax but don't just lie on the sofa. Go out for a long walk to increase your circulation, do some mild exercise to purge the toxins but don't work too hard, just enough to give you a bit of a glow. Once you have had some fresh air, then you have earned the right to some time in a comfortable chair with a good film or book – or even the Sunday papers.

Have a relaxing lavender bath before bed and try to get an early night. The lavender bath relaxes both body and mind – it is also a key ingredient in the Weekend Detox but can provide some much needed support here as well. Lavender essential oil is brilliant for the Quick-Fix Hangover Detox as its main properties are those of calming, soothing and balancing. Balancing is the key: detox is about bringing life into balance, getting rid of the bad and enhancing the good, removing the stress and adding the calm. In a balanced state we can mend. Mind, body and spirit are all given a chance to heal if they are no longer under pressure.

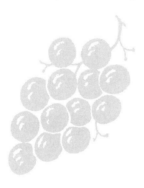

There is nothing more likely to put you out of balance than a corker of a hangover. Bathing in lavender will ease muscle tension, encourage cell growth, balance your mood, and relax you in preparation for a much-needed night's sleep. By the time you wake you should be clear of any alcoholic residue and hopefully you will have made up your sleep deficit from the day before.

Never again . . .

3 The Healthy Mind Detox

The Healthy Mind Detox takes you through 10 days and 10 tasks. Each day you carry out a task that makes you look at yourself, your life or your thoughts differently. Getting a new perspective gives you the chance to see if you are getting what you want and need out of your life. If you can think clearly then problems seem easier to solve. You can come to a decision more quickly if you just keep to the salient points.

Following the Healthy Mind Detox programme actually requires you to stop and take a really long look, not just at yourself but inside yourself and all around yourself. Remember, the whole programme can be completely private. You may wish to write things down on a day-to-day basis, or you may wish to Healthy Mind Detox by simply using your mind.

Part of looking at yourself is being truthful about what you want in life: not just health, wealth and happiness (join the queue!), but much more specific things, things that can be done immediately. Keeping your eye on the big picture is very important but you also have to have the smaller, more immediate pictures coloured in to keep you going.

You will be asked to think about what you really desire.

Desire is better than want because it injects a real passion and passion is a strong motivational tool. Do you desire to live in the house you live in? Do you desire to landscape the garden? Do you desire more friends or fewer friends? Do you desire to go out more? etc, etc. If you sort out the small picture desires then the big picture comes into focus quite naturally.

PREPARATION TIPS

Live for the moment

Future planning is very, very important but don't wish your life away! Living for the moment is great fun. You get loads more out of each day without doing anything other than living your life and feeling how it feels. Living for the moment means thinking for the moment. Think about things you can do today, today. And leave thinking about things you cannot do until tomorrow until tomorrow.

If you don't organise your brain this way then, before you know it, you will be thinking about everything at every moment during your day and never actually get on with 'doing' anything! How easy is it, when you have an exciting weekend booked, to spend Monday, Tuesday, Wednesday, Thursday and Friday thinking about Saturday? Poor weekdays, what did they ever do to deserve being wished away? Saturday and Sunday were always guaranteed – they weren't going anywhere – so why not enjoy the weekdays *and* the weekend. You should also learn to waste time deliberately. Let your mind relax and regenerate, actually plan to do nothing, do things for no reason but don't just let time slip away unnoticed – use it as relaxation so that when you want to think about something you are ready to.

Get rid of mental clutter

Our minds are fantastic at holding information and that's very important for day-to-day life. But we are also good at holding on to things we don't need, both physically and, more importantly, mentally. We bear grudges, we get niggled that someone has something we don't, we get annoyed that the bus didn't arrive on time yesterday, we worry that the bus won't even come on Thursday and so on and so on. Healthy Mind Detox will look at ways to sort out the things you can do something about – and make you do them. It will also sort out the things you cannot do anything about and make you forget them, or file them safely to be dealt with at a more suitable time. Worrying about something that may never happen, or has happened, is exhausting and wastes energy. *Doing* something to stop you worrying is exhilarating and a much better use of your time.

Be true to yourself

The only way to be true to yourself is to know who is the real you. What does your mind think about your body? What do *you* think about your mind? What do *you* think about your body? Are they all the same? Or do you separate them? Do you 'feel' or do you 'do'? Are you what other people think you are or is there another side that hasn't been let out for fear of shocking them? Or do you deliberately go out of your way to cause a stir? Can you change the bits you don't want and enhance the bits you really like?

Every one of these tasks will help you understand and discover something about yourself. Once you have completed the tasks, you will know yourself, know how you feel, know what you want in life and how to go about getting it. You will know how to just do stuff, to live in the moment, know how to clear out your personal junk, and how to keep hold of the bits you like and use them to your advantage.

It will feel so good that you will be desperately keen to try out the 'New Improved You'.

But it won't be easy. There will be days when you feel exhausted because you will be using your mind in a way that it hasn't been used for years. A breath of fresh air always makes you more tired but a healthy tired, not the tiredness born of boredom. Clearing your mind will stop you worrying unnecessarily and stop you stressing over things that may never actually become reality. A detoxed mind is clear of everything but the essential or enjoyable.

So follow this plan to bring a smile to your face and a feel-good factor into your life.

CHECK LIST

Detoxing your mind requires a little preparation. You will need:

- a notebook
- a pen
- something technical that you have never truly mastered
- some writing paper
- relaxing music or a relaxation tape
- a local telephone directory or information brochure of clubs and associations
- local newspapers for a couple of weeks
- bus and train timetables
- your imagination
- your open mind . . .

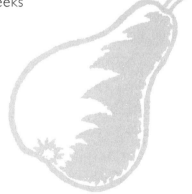

THE 10 DAYS AND 10 TASKS

Day 1:	Smile
Day 2:	Learn a technical function
Day 3:	Create some space in your head
Day 4:	Inject some creativity into your life
Day 5:	Talk to yourself
Day 6:	Take a perceived risk
Day 7:	Let yourself daydream
Day 8:	Spend time, not money
Day 9:	Retreat into silence
Day 10:	Write your personal cosmic shopping list

DAY 1: SMILE

It is said that children smile an average of 400 times a day, whilst adults only manage to crack a grin 15 times a day.

It's a shame that something so simple sometimes seems so hard. We get out of the habit of smiling because there is so much else to think about, so much else that is serious and doesn't warrant a smile. But, if you look at it the other way, it would be so much better to do the serious stuff with a smile. If you are asking someone to do something then smiling makes the task seem much easier and more fun. And if you smile when doing a task, the task seems somehow lighter, less arduous.

If we meet someone with a 'friendly' smile or a 'happy' smile then it's hard not to smile back; it makes us feel good too. If we have a laugh or something makes us giggle then everything becomes less difficult, less problematic.

So today, Day 1 of your programme, you should think about your smile:

- Smile at your neighbour and say good morning or hello with a big smile.

- The first person you meet in the street, say hello with a smile.

- When you pick up the phone, say your number or name with a smile.

- If anyone opens a door for you then say thank you and smile.

- If you need to read anything or go through a document then make sure you exchange that dour, serious look for a smile – it will make the read that much more interesting.

- Write your diary with a smile. Think of all the fabulous things you have done and the people you have met. Smile and a normal everyday task becomes a joy.

Smiling is catching, it is contagious, there is nothing more likely to make you giggle than somone who is giggling uncontrollably themselves. There is nothing more likely to make you smile than someone giving you a great big grin. Find something on a daily basis that will let you have a little chuckle to yourself.

The main thing to remember with smiling is that you have to mean it. If you sit in front of a mirror first thing in the morning or during the evening of the day before your 'smile-in' and simply make the shape of a smile you will see that it looks awful. You will also recognise it as the sort of smile you get from tired shop assistants or from someone who truly doesn't want to smile but feels that they have to at least look a bit happier. No, smiling needs to be meant, a real smile will light up your face, crinkle your eyes and wrinkle your nose, it will show your teeth and lift your cheeks and it will make you feel great. So try a few out, mainly to remind yourself just how good you look when wearing a smile, and then you are fully prepared for the day ahead.

Top tips

The smile must be genuine.

Keep a diary. Write down a few words about how you felt about smiling all day. Was it exhausting or uplifting? Did it feel strange at first or did it feel natural? Did you enjoy it?

Did it make you smile?

DAY 2: LEARN A TECHNICAL FUNCTION

Get out the manual and get to grips with it once and for all time . . .

Choose an appliance that you have never really understood how to use. For instance:

- The video recorder
- The deep-fat fryer, the juicer, the food processor – watch those fingers
- The memory on the telephone
- The delicates wash on your machine
- Storing names on your mobile phone
- Setting up an ansaphone service on your mobile phone
- Checking the oil and water in the engine of your car
- Setting the timer in your central heating thermostat
- Learning to wire a plug
- Programming the padlock on your suitcase

Once you have chosen your appliance, choose a function that has always been pushed to the back of your mind or, alternatively, has always been labelled as someone else's job – and quite simply, teach yourself how to do it. The manual will take you through it step by step. And if at first you don't succeed, just breathe deeply and try again.

Top tips

Make sure you have all the relevant parts described in the manual. If a vital piece is missing or broken, you will find it very hard to get any results and this will be very unsatisfying indeed.

Make sure you find something you want to solve. If you never use the video or never need to put the oven on timer then there will be little satisfaction in learning the process. Choose to programme your telephone instead, with all your most often used numbers.

Make a mental note of how your task will make your life easier and less complicated:

- You can watch more programmes as you can now record important programmes that clash for later.

- You can do more chores on Sundays and still enjoy a full Sunday roast.

- You can call your friends and tell them all your news without searching for your address book first.

- You won't need to pull into a service station during a long journey to replenish water for your windscreen. More importantly, you will never run out of oil and ruin your engine.

- You can come home to a wonderfully warm house in the middle of winter.

- You can open your suitcase secure in the knowledge that it still holds its original contents.

Make a mental note of other things you could do in the technical field to make your life easier – and make a date to do them.

DAY 3: CREATE SOME SPACE IN YOUR HEAD

We all have ghosts or skeletons in our minds. We are full of 'what if', 'I wonder', 'should have' and 'if only'.

If we used this time more effectively, doing something about our worries instead of just worrying, then we would clear a lot more space and create a lot more peace in our minds.

Because we believe there is nothing we can do to sort out the situation, we keep going over and over it in our minds and using valuable space that would be better used for something positive and constructive.

Today we can clean the thoughts away or file them so that they can be used when we *choose* to use them, rather than springing to mind when we least need them to.

The first step is to note down all the things that:

- You truly believe you cannot do anything about but want to, in order to clear them out of your thoughts.

- You constantly think about and want to do something about.

Now you can start to make amends and clear your mind. Taking the situations and individuals one at a time, write them a letter. Make sure that you cover every issue that concerns you and make sure that you put in the letter exactly how you feel about the situation. Include anything that has resulted from this situation or incident and any repercussions that have occurred since then. Take every thought that creeps into your mind and put it down on paper.

Whatever you decide to do with these letters (store them, burn them, read them or even send them), you can rest assured that all your unsettled business is now settled. All your thoughts have been faced – they won't have gone away but they have now been managed and you should feel really positive that you have taken some action.

In future make sure you 'sort' your thoughts before they get too disruptive. If you can say what you feel, say it right on the spot so that it doesn't fester. If you don't want to say it then write a letter immediately and send it. The sooner you write, the less you will have to say because you haven't had time to dwell on it and make a mountain out of a molehill. But *do* think before you write as, once it has been sent, it has been said!

Writing your thoughts down in a letter enables you to say anything to anyone, any time. The sooner you get your thoughts down on paper, the sooner they stop spinning round in your head.

Day 4: Inject some creativity into your life

Do something different, swap things around and see how it feels. Get a new perspective.

- I get up at the same time
- I have the same thing for breakfast
- I go into my office
- I have lunch
- I finish at the same time every day
- I go home
- I watch TV
- I make supper
- I go to bed
- I get up at the same time . . .

Sounds familiar?

There is no room in there for any creativity. I know what happens and when it happens during my day, so I have no need to think about anything because it just happens that way! Now, if I was to change everything around – I would need to keep my wits about me in order to get everything done in the same length of time.

Your day of change should be total. Everything you do should be done differently. Choose a day that would have been completely routine and turn it topsy turvy:

- Set the alarm earlier or later
- Get out of the other side of the bed
- Have your shower/bath before breakfast or after breakfast, whichever is not the norm
- Wear a completely different outfit. If you normally wear dark colours then choose anything you have that is bright and vice versa. Wear trousers not skirts. Wear ties not bow ties. Wear cufflinks. Carry a handbag not a carry-all
- If you normally wear make-up then go fresh-faced
- If you don't wear aftershave then put some on
- Get the bus instead of taking the car, or take the car instead of the train
- Buy tea on the way into work rather than coffee
- Take the stairs, not the lifts
- If you normally have tea then use herbal or make coffee instead
- If you normally go to lunch then buy a sandwich to eat at your desk or bring in a packed lunch
- If you call your friends in the afternoon then call them in the morning
- Leave work later than normal or go earlier
- Go a different route home
- Eat out if you normally eat in, or cook something that you have never had before or get a friend to cook
- Watch TV if you normally read, or read if you usually watch TV
- Call your parents today instead of Friday

- Do the weekly shop late evening instead of Saturday morning
- Have a bath before you go to bed or take a shower
- Read a book or talk about the day instead of going straight to sleep
- Apply moisturiser if you don't normally, then turn off the light.

Any of the above activities could make you look at your day completely differently. You may want to change things permanently, or you may decide to go back to normal. It's up to you. But, for today, be different, be refreshing and inspiring.

DAY 5: TALK TO YOURSELF

Today you must take time out to get to know your 'self'. You may think this is an odd idea. Surely you know everything about your 'self' that there is to know? This is true. But, as with anything familiar, you probably take your 'self' for granted.

Every day you carry out tasks, jobs and roles. But how do you really feel about them? Have you listened to how your body feels? And do you know how you really feel about your diet, your figure, your mind, your exercise regime, your daily routine, etc., etc.

What I mean about talking to yourself is really listening to yourself and then finding a response – starting a dialogue. We do lots of things that, if we took time to listen to our own response, we would not do or we would do differently. If someone calls and says they need your help to look after their children for a day – you immediately say 'Yes, no problem.' If you stopped to think and listen to yourself you may have found that you have a very busy day and it would suit you better if you jointly decided on a solution/date/entertainment for all the kids that meant everyone was happy.

If you think you need to go to the gym to keep fit then you pack a bag and toddle off to your next work-out. But if you listened to your body you might find that it would rather wait until tomorrow. Your muscles will have had time to recover from yesterday's workout and your mind will be much more energetic. Exercise *now* would be a trial – something you had to get through – but exercise *tomorrow* would be invigorating and a great tonic.

(NB: Listening to yourself should not be an excuse never to do the things you hate, but need to do!!! If you really listened you would know they had to be done.)

Listening to yourself should also give you a much more in-depth understanding of how you feel about yourself. For the Healthy Mind Detox programme you need to start to listen to yourself in a slightly different way, a way that will get you into the habit of listening thoroughly in the future. You need to start writing to yourself – it really works and the letters will amaze you.

Write a letter to yourself about how you feel. Here's an example . . .

I am really looking forward to the weekend but it seems as if I just get to Friday, collapse because I am tired and, before I know it, it is Sunday evening again – without me even noticing the weekend.

It would be nice to cancel everything and just rest. I know the pressure is to get things done, but sooner or later getting things done will turn into bare survival. I am tired and need to make time for me.

Once you have written to yourself you should always give your body a chance to respond. This was the response that the individual felt her body would write as a result of receiving the letter above:

> This is good. I do need a rest but you don't need to stop everything.
> What I would really enjoy is a session in a beauty salon – pedicure,
> manicure, bikini line – and top it all off with a glass of wine and a nice
> takeaway . . . Then I will be refreshed and feel as if I actually spent time
> on me.

The result was that the relentless tussle she was having, between enjoying herself and not becoming exhausted, was simply resolved by taking the time to find out what would actually replenish her stocks.

This meant that there was loads of space in her life to get on with other things – she had cleared the fug out of her head.

Before you start

You will need a quiet, warm room for an hour and a pad and pen. You may like to have a tape of relaxation music – make sure it is only music as lyrics are likely to interfere with your thoughts. Alternatively your relaxation tape may have a relaxation exercise sequence on it. In that case, you can simply follow the tape. If not, then follow the sequence below or refer to the relaxation sequence in the User's Manual (pp. 170–2).

Today you will be writing a broad-ranging letter, a letter that says to your 'self' how you are feeling, what you want, what's causing you concern, and what is good – basically anything that is currently going round in your mind.

In order to get the best out of 'Talking to yourself' you should always precede your session with a relaxation exercise. The whole process should take you no more than an hour but it is important to include the relaxation as you will get much more out of it.

RELAXATION AND DEEP BREATHING

- Lie in a comfortable position, with your back flat to the floor/bed/mat. Or, if you have back problems, place a cushion under your thighs and knees and this will naturally support your back.

- Place your arms loosely by your sides and let your legs flop open. Make sure your shoulders are relaxed and your neck straight.
- To ensure everything is relaxed, start by scrunching every muscle in your body as tightly as possible, hold it for a count of four and then let everything relax into the floor.
- To make sure that you are breathing correctly, simply relax your stomach muscles, inhale through your nose slowly and take in the air until it feels as if the base of your stomach is full of air.
- Pause momentarily and then exhale through the mouth.
- When you can feel the air 'in your stomach' it shows you have relaxed your diaphragm muscle, which means your lungs have fully expanded and you have inhaled to full capacity. This may feel strange at first but it should soon become the normal way to breathe and you won't need to think about it any more.

Writing your letter to yourself

Now take your pen and write a letter to yourself. Be very honest. If you feel bad put all that in, and if you feel good put all that in. If you like something then say so and if you hate something then say so. Don't try and interpret how you are feeling; just tell it like it is. Remember – no one will ever see this letter. It is *yours*.

Once you have completed your letter, sit back, do some breathing and then read it back to yourself slowly. The letter will deserve a response. Write back and say how you feel after reading the letter. How do you feel about it? Did it surprise you or shock you? Did you find out about feelings you didn't know you had?

Having completed today's task you will be different. You will have found out more about yourself, you will have cleared out the things you now know to be irrelevant, and you will have kept the things you have decided are important. You won't have solved all your problems but you will have seen them all from a new perspective . . .

Relax. Do not try to change things. We are working at a pace that is natural and we will get there in our own time. Let the fluctuations go by, let the bad equal the good, don't 'need more control' – I am happy that we are working together – I am happy that whatever comes is not right or wrong. I will listen more to your requests and signals without stressing or trying to change them . . .

DAY 6: TAKE A PERCEIVED RISK

Test your comfort zone and feel the thrill.

If anything concentrates the mind it is a small dose of abject terror! Not only does it concentrate the mind but, as you go through the 'my whole life flashed before me' bit, you also get to take a long look at yourself and that is incredibly interesting. You find out so much about yourself and how you feel, how you react, in just a few small moments.

Now, Healthy Mind Detox is not about putting you at risk – far from it. But it *is* about looking at things differently in order to clear your mind of the rubbish and keep the important stuff. Putting yourself through an extreme experience (with all safety measures observed so there is no *actual* risk) is a very good way to find out what is important to you.

Perceived risks can be taken by going along to a place where there are professionals ready and equipped to take you through an extreme experience whilst observing all the correct safety rules and guidelines. They will also assess if you are fit and able to carry out the task without putting yourself in any danger. The risk is all in your head!

The sorts of things we are talking about are:

- Parachute jumping
- Rock climbing
- Flying
- White-water rafting
- Going on a balloon flight
- Going on a glider
- Holding an insect or reptile
- Mountain biking
- Cave diving
- Bidding at an auction
- Scuba diving
- Public speaking

The list goes on . . . It is hard to name everything that would fit into this category but you need to find something that would truly be a massive thing for you to do.

Top tips

Just because something is a big deal for you does not mean it would be such a big deal for the next person. Just do something that would really challenge you. Don't listen to anyone else about what they think would be the most terrifying thing. Work it out for yourself and then, when you feel ready, start to make the necessary arrangements.

Call the association or club that operates the 'risk of your choice' and find out as much as you feel you need to know.

Once you have found something that you would like to have a go at, and that fits your budget and your timing, then just book it!

Obviously this is a lot to get done in one day but you should be able to start to think through the project – and work out the best time to schedule your risk taking. Good luck and fingers crossed!

If you can do this – is there anything beyond your reach?

DAY 7: LET YOURSELF DAYDREAM

Today you have permission to daydream about anything you want to. You can think about all the things you wish for and all the things you dream about. Today is a total release from the real world. You can wish for *anything*.

Start by writing down ten wishes or dreams. As with everything on this programme, they must be totally personal and can be very selfish. But they must be things that are currently in your head, things that you sometimes mull over in your mind during the day.

Your dreams and wishes should be your real dreams and wishes. For instance:

- I want to sing with Frank Sinatra/Elvis
- I want to fly to the moon
- I want to fly around the world in a hot-air balloon
- I want to be 6 foot tall
- I want an IQ of 2,000
- I want to rule the world

Once you have the list then just sit back and enjoy it. Imagine yourself ruling the world – shortly after winning *Mastermind*. Tickets to the moon in your back pocket and the roar of the crowd still fresh in your mind from last nights concert with Elvis. Waiting to hear from the palace for an appointment to measure up for your crown. Feels good, doesn't it? And I bet you at least have a smile on your face, if you haven't laughed out loud.

In your mind you can be and do anything you want. So go ahead! Dream on and wish away.

Now that you have got into the swing of it you can get on with your normal day and transform it into the most amazing day you have ever had – a 'DAY-DREAM'. Everything you do today will be the stuff that dreams are made of.

> Leave your palace early in the morning to travel to the Mastermind studios. On your way, help some university students with their dissertations.
>
> Give Elvis some hints and tips on being successful as a pop star. Meet up with some old friends for lunch and decide to take the whole afternoon off in order to shop for everything you have ever wanted. When you have picked the children up from school you will be going to see Mickey Mouse who has called to say that he has a spare hour or so and can he come and entertain the children whilst you prepare the sumptuous evening meal.
>
> After the meal the children say they want to go to bed as they are tired, and you and your partner fly off to the coast in your hot-air balloon to see the sunset. Once you return you can pay the babysitter and go to bed – to awake to a breakfast of fresh fruit salad in a champagne juice with poached eggs on light French toast . . . Get the picture?

You see, I have everything and anything I want, every day of my life. I just dream for 5 minutes and there it all is – it doesn't cost a penny and it feels soooooo good.

'Dreamers' and 'people who wish their life away', are usually considered to be rather hopeless: people who have no real aim in life or who cannot come to terms with reality. But if they know that they are dreaming or wishing and they are happy to return to the real world refreshed, having had a little entertainment and excitement, then I think dreamers and wishers are probably the only people who do have any real idea of what is going on. They are aware of the real world and also of their own very personal world – the world of their own minds. And everyone knows that, if you know your own mind, you can do anything.

DAY 8: SPEND TIME, NOT MONEY

If we wake up and think 'what should I/we do today', one of the major considerations is how much money we've got. If we have a lot, at the start of the month, then we have more choice than the end of the month when funds are running low. If we have no money we tend to think we cannot do anything, and if we have had a windfall or a win on the lottery(!) then we can do absolutely anything.

Yet having money sometimes stops us thinking about all the options we have. We tend to ignore the simple, straightforward options and go for the more complicated. We have learnt that you can only have fun if you have money. This is not true. If we put in a bit more thought and use our heads, there are millions of things we can do to keep occupied, learn new things or entertain ourselves, that cost nothing.

For one whole day on this programme (during a weekend or holiday) you are going to detox your mind of all the short cuts to happiness, and actually think about how to spend your time without spending any money.

This has not been dropped on you without any preparation – the check list on p. 67 includes keeping the local papers that are delivered to your house for the weeks preceding your detox, the local bus timetable and train timetable. This is where they come into their own. It may also be worth checking out the local post office window, local council offices, local social centre and the local sports centre noticeboard.

You will need to collect all these sources of information together. Then all you need is £5 per adult and £3 per child, and your imagination.

The money is really only for emergencies – you win extra points if you do not spend anything during the day.

To begin with here is a list of activities that are no longer permitted, because they will cost money or won't use any form of imagination or brainpower. If you never think about how you use your time then it will just slip away. You will be old before your time and you won't have anything to show for it.

- Television
- Cinema
- Dining out
- Shopping
- Holidays
- Driving anywhere
- Meeting friends for coffee
- Buying ice creams
- Going to the leisure centre
- Pub lunch

The following activities cost nothing and are very definitely permitted:

- Having a long bath, relaxing and doing lots of home beauty treatments (e.g. tea bags on eyes, cucumber on eyes, salt scrubs, cold showers)
- Making a cake/having friends for dinner/having friends for lunch using foods from the cupboard
- Weeding the garden
- Going for a walk or hiking around your town/area
- Tidying out a room/cupboard
- Looking around a local church/museum/gallery that has free entrance

- Checking local papers for outdoor craft fairs to look round – not buying!
- Attending talks at the local town hall that may be going on for no entrance fee
- Finding out where your local library is and going and reading about anything you wish to
- Doing a day of voluntary work
- Sorting out all your old clothes and delivering them to a local charity shop
- Putting all your photographs into your album or at least sorting them out and throwing away all the shots that are out of focus or too dark
- Reading a book
- Visting a friend you haven't seen in ages but who lives in walking distance
- Sewing buttons on to everything that has lost a button but you never get round to doing it

And so on. In fact the list of things that cost nothing is much longer and much more interesting than the list of things that cost a lot!

Top tips

Try not to prepare too much. Collect the papers and timetables but don't look at them until the morning of your chosen day. This will mean that you have to use your mind more to come up with something interesting or productive to do.

If you think about the day too much in advance you may inadvertently get things into the house that will help you entertain yourself – the challenge is to come up with things on the spur of the moment – a genuine case of 'what shall I do today?'.

Try to remain as sociable as normal. Don't think that you have to be lonely just because you have no funds. Encourage your friends to join your challenge. They should be your entertainment, not just people that you spend money with.

Make a mental note of how you react to having no funds available. Is it unnerving or a challenge? Do you talk more to friends whilst walking or meeting than you normally do or is it the same? Do you look at things differently? Is it more tiring having to use your mind to entertain yourself or is it more uplifting? Have you got things done that have been hanging around for ever, or did you use your time to try out totally new things?

Ask yourself if you will try this again in the future, or do you think the way you spend your spare time is fulfilling enough?

Are you using money instead of imagination?

DAY 9: RETREAT INTO SILENCE

Today should be a day off work, a weekend or a holiday, as you will spend it in total silence.

Getting to know what is in your head, what you are thinking, how you are reacting, is very easy if you are not interacting with anyone. If the only dialogue you have all day is with yourself then you can find out a lot. It's like being locked in a room with one person and you are free to ask any question you wish. It may be very telling and quite intense. And you will get answers to many of your questions.

There are many places that call themselves 'retreats'. These are places where people – often religious – can go to stay for a time of reflection or prayer. You do not enter into conversation with anyone on retreat so you can remain focused on your reasons for being there. You can create these retreat surroundings in your own home and spend your time thinking for yourself: writing lists; writing letters; and sorting things out, physically, emotionally or mentally.

You will need to prepare for this day by shutting yourself off from the outside world and any outside stimuli. Put the ansaphone on or unplug the phone. Lock the front door and do not answer it, do not open the post. There will be no radio or television, no videos, no newspapers, no books. Make sure the day is a full 24 hours, from say 11 p.m. the night before until 11 p.m. on the day of your retreat. Many of these hours will be whilst you are asleep. Indeed, if you use your retreat day to catch up on lost sleep then that is very useful.

Dress in something loose, warm and comfortable but make sure you do dress. If you need to catch up on sleep then sleep in until you wake. Get up and dressed and if you need more sleep then go back to bed for rest as and when required during the day. For the rest of your retreat time you should try to avoid your normal activities. Don't try to do all the household chores and catch up with tidying the house. Retreat should be about you – the whole 10 days should be about you. Retreat means touching base with yourself.

This may be the first day that you have truly spent on your own. Even though you may normally spend a lot of time on your own, the rule of silence makes you think about yourself more. Use the day to answer any questions you have for yourself. If you have any problems with relationships, use the time to think through all your options. If you need to decide about your job – not about a problem at work – but about yourself in the context of work – then think this through. The fact that you cannot communicate with the outside world means that, if you reach a decision, you will have to live with that decision for several hours before you tell anyone. This may give you more time to reflect and to confirm if the decision is right or wrong for you. If there is a lot going on in your life then your day of silence may simply serve to 'let contents settle' before you carry on with business as usual. We file thoughts in our head so that we can access them at a later date; this important filing process can take place when you are relaxing.

If you believe that you are very straight and organised in your head, and that there is nothing you would like time to think through, then well done. What's your secret!? Seriously, even if you have everything sorted, you should still 'retreat' and use the time for deep relaxation exercises, correct breathing and doing nothing. Doing nothing is extremely hard: listen to your breathing, feel your heart beat through your body and become aware of every aspect of your mind and body. When they are in total harmony, prepare a simple meal of cleansing food from the food lists in the User's Manual (see pp. 160–3) and get an early night. You may find that after relaxation your dreams are very much more vivid as your brain goes through its own subconscious sorting process.

Top tips

Remember, you must not do anything that involves any outside stimuli. Retreat is about you and your own mind – no books, no papers, no conversation (except in your own head), no words, no television, no radio, no magazines.

A good view out of the window of the country, sky or garden – no streets or people – is all you are permitted. If the views from your retreat include traffic or people then look inwards at your own house and cut off the outside world. If something distracts you just let it pass, don't dwell on it, and return to your own thoughts.

Awake feeling refreshed, invigorated and clear-headed after your day of silence.

Day 10: Write your personal cosmic shopping list

Having a personal cosmic shopping list is like looking into the future and seeing just how you will be when you have achieved everything you want to achieve. A personal cosmic shopping list means you can be where you want to be, at any time.

As with everything in the Healthy Mind Detox programme your cosmic shopping list is personal and should apply to yourself, for yourself. Your list should be easy to remember and include everything you can envisage yourself having.

Your list can include yourself or others and it should be positive; nothing negative should be on your list. You don't want to think yourself into a negative situation.

Write what you want in life, and where you want to be, and eventually you will get there. For instance:

- I have a successful profitable business
- I have done everything I want to for my family at this time
- I am rested and ready to move forward
- I have a lot of time for myself
- I have started a new hobby that really inspires me
- My relationship is better now than it has been. We seem to grow closer together as each year passes
- I have loads of confidence . . .

You get the picture – simple but clearly describing yourself as you want to be, but in the present tense. A self-fulfilling prophecy.

Well done. You now have a crystal-clear picture of where you are going and how good it feels. Simply go there in your mind and it will become reality quicker than you imagine . . .

4 The Weekend Detox

Short detox programmes are not something I usually believe in, generally because the 'short' often stands for 'short cut' or 'cheat'. Detox programmes where you are asked to do nothing other than mix a strange potion from a bottle or simply add a few vegetables to your current diet are not good. They will at best have no effect; at worst they could upset your digestion and put you off detox altogether. However, the following 48-hour plan will give your body a real break. It will let you see just how good you can feel, and it will show you that detoxing really is worthwhile.

So, on one of those rare occasions when you find you have 48 hours to concentrate on number one, lock the doors, put the ansaphone on and switch off the mobile. This two-day plan will transform you from a tired and worn-out 'human doing' on Friday afternoon to a revitalised, refreshed and regenerated 'human being' on Monday morning. Of course, if you have time off during the week, you can just adjust the days, e.g. Tuesday evening through to Friday morning.

Create your own home spa with the Weekend Detox and you will feel amazing. Slough your way to svelte, smooth limbs and streamline yourself to sleek, toned slenderness and get a flat stomach to boot. Detox can be pure indulgence – no, really – massage, aromatherapy, exfoliation, wraps, rubs and relaxation. All of these can purge you of unwanted toxins and promote internal healing and external fabulousness.

Enrol some friends but make sure you are totally dedicated to the stunning new you. No one else matters – this is your time to make *you* feel great.

There is a lot to do. As with any weekend away, you will need to plan, prepare and pack – well, put out ready to use. The weekend is designed to make you feel as if you have been truly whisked away to an oasis of calm and comfort, to be pampered back to health and vitality. In order to feel like your break is just a moment away I have taken the liberty of sending you the schedule for your 48-hour stay. Read on . . .

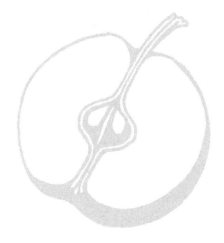

SCHEDULE

EVENING I

8.30p.m. Arrive

Lavender bath

Early night with diary

DAY I

Awake to a refreshing cup of lemon juice and hot water

Shower to wash away the week – no need to wash your hair

Dress in loose, comfortable clothing

Have breakfast, choosing from fresh fruits, juices, smoothies
and tisanes

Rest in 'relaxation lounge', reading good book or magazines

Prepare for reflexology treatment

Mid-morning snack, choosing from fresh fruit, a selection of nuts
or home-made muesli

Yoga stretch

Rest in 'relaxation lounge' prior to lunch

Lunch of grilled fish or goat's cheese roulade, fragrant rice and
freshly tossed green salad

Country walk to indulge the senses

Meditation

Head wrap and scalp massage

Relaxation – reading or watching a film

6.30 p.m. Supper of Thai vegetable soup and spicy vegetable grill

Dry 'float relax'

Natural manicure and hand massage

9.30 p.m. Sleep and recover

DAY 2

Rise

Hot water and lemon juice

Refreshing walk to open your eyes to the world

Stretch and relax

Exfoliating scrub, thermotherapy bath and body drench

Relaxation session in 'relaxation lounge' with lymph drainage

Light lunch of tisanes and assorted grapes

Time for reading, writing in your diary, or reflection

List writing and right-drawer compilation

Candle meditation or 20-minute snooze break

Prepare for friends arriving

6.30 p.m. Light supper for friends, partner or family

Early night

MORNING 3

Arise, breakfast of non-dairy yogurt and home-made nut and seed muesli

Emerge refreshed, renewed and '48-hour' detoxed.

You see, it sounds fabulous and does you good. If you look carefully there are several tried-and-tested tools for 'heavy-duty detox'. But the programme is so user-friendly that you won't realise just how strict you are being on yourself.

Look and see if you can spot the 24-hour mini fast, the mini Detox Yourself food programme, the hydrotherapy and the mini, mini Mind Detox. All in a day's work – but it will leave you feeling wonderful and thoroughly cleansed.

As there are several very serious reasons to do the 48-hour detox, there is a full explanatory section in the User's Manual at the back of the book (see pp. 187–91). The manual contains full details of fasts and mini fasts and why they are good for you. Please read this section thoroughly before you go ahead, to gain a better understanding of the good you are doing to your body, both inside and out.

Preparation lists

Even though the programme is just 48 hours, you will need to do some serious preparation. Taking it easy is the key and having everything to hand makes taking it easy even easier.

Equipment

- Tidy rooms: bedroom, lounge, kitchen and bathroom (nothing to distract you into tidying up!)
- Warm rooms – put the heating up a notch, as you will be wearing a dressing gown and loose clothing for 48 hours, or make sure you have the materials to light a cosy fire in the rooms you are in
- Lavender essential oil
- A citrus or floral oil of your choice
- Olive oil
- A diary or note pad
- Pens and pencil and/or crayons
- Freshly washed dressing gown, housecoat or warm pyjamas
- Freshly made bed with crisp, clean sheets/covers
- Somewhere to sit with your feet up, e.g. a sofa with cushions, an armchair with a footstool or a day bed
- A duvet or rug

- Selection of reading material – to your taste but nothing work-related
- Sunflower oil or any base oil, grapeseed, sweet almond, etc
- Clean fluffy towels (hand and bath size)
- A route to walk from your home or flat
- Exfoliating product, glove, mitt or moisturiser with natural sea salt
- Lots of pillows
- Candles, night-lites or just a selection of normal candles
- Relaxing music

Food

- Fresh unwaxed lemons
- Assorted fresh fruit
- Assorted herbal teas or your favourite herbal tea
- Portion of oily fish or goat's or sheep's cheese
- Short-grain brown rice
- Olive oil
- Mixed fresh vegetables
- Lots of water – tap or bottled (bottled is best)
- Lots of grapes
- Vegetarian stock – low-salt or no-salt
- Lemongrass
- Chillies
- Goat's yoghurt
- A selection of nuts and seeds (e.g. hazelnuts, Brazil nuts, walnuts, and sunflower, caraway and sesame seeds)

Full food lists are included in the User's Manual (see pp. 160–4). Choose from these foods to create your chosen evening menu for your Weekend Detox, and do your shopping as required.

The programme details

The Weekend Detox programme is obviously designed to be carried out over a weekend. This is because many people can take weekends off, with no work or family commitments. But there is no reason why the programme shouldn't be done at absolutely any time – just find 48 hours and off you go. Start one evening and go through to the evening two days later. By being good at breakfast on the third day you can also complete a full 52-hour programme for not much extra effort but huge gain – go on!

Evening 1

Starting at 8.30 p.m. effectively allows you to go home, change, pack, travel and arrive, ready to detox. Starting at 6.30 p.m. will mean a mad dash to be ready and arriving somewhat dishevelled. Get home from work or being out, change into comfortable 'weekend' clothing, and finish all vital odd chores and tasks.

If you have a partner and/or kids, arrange for them to go away for the weekend. Then:

- Have a light supper
- Tidy up the rooms you will be using
- Plug in the ansaphone
- Arrange for friends who are doing the programme with you to arrive by 8 p.m. for a relaxed start
- 'Check them into' their rooms (i.e. put the sleeping bags on the mattresses!)
- Do anything that will make the next 48 hours more relaxing
- Check the hot water is on and that there is enough

- Check the heating is on if required
- Take a deep breath – and sink into the calm of detox . . .

The lavender bath

At 8.30 p.m. we should be winding down from the week or the last few days; we should have eaten at least an hour ago so that our bodies have time to digest and process our food before we go to bed. In reality, this hardly ever happens. If we are lucky enough to be home from work then we are more likely to be bathing the kids or putting them to bed. If we have older kids we are probably waiting around to be the taxi service, or we're just catching up on everything we haven't had time to do earlier.

The lavender bath relaxes both body and mind. Lavender essential oil is brilliant for starting a detox programme, as its main properties are those of calming, soothing and balancing. Detox is about bringing life into balance, getting rid of the bad and enhancing the good, removing the stress and adding the calm. In a balanced state we can mend. Mind, body and spirit are all given a chance to heal if they are no longer under pressure. Bathing in lavender will ease muscle tension, encourage cell regrowth, balance your mood and relax you, in preparation for a wonderful, full night's sleep. Lavender is also one of the safest oils. Very few people have a negative reaction to it and, if small amounts are inadvertently applied neat to the skin, it will not burn.

Please see the instructions for preparing your bath in the User's Manual (pp. 178–9).

Early night with diary

You should be tucked up in bed by 9.30 p.m. at the latest.

Slip into your freshly made bed and feel the cool of the sheets warm up from the heat of your lavender bath . . . Feels good, doesn't it?

This not only means you get a wonderfully early night but it gives your body time to relax physically and emotionally for a full 12 hours.

Sleep is a great healer in itself, and – after your lavender bath – you should have created the ideal conditions for a night's deep sleep. Lavender has powerful sedative qualities and will help in almost all cases of insomnia, not least because it calms an over-active brain.

Writing in your diary or note pad will help you to detox all the unwanted thoughts that spin around your mind preventing you from relaxing mentally. Write down everything you are thinking.

If you are worried, writing will help you to 'see' the problem and give you a fresh perspective.

If you are busy, writing will mean you have put everything down on paper so you will not be able to forget anything.

If you are happy, writing will allow you to keep that positive feeling for longer. If you find yourself unhappy at a later date, you can re-read your diary and remember the good times.

You can write to yourself and tell yourself good news – how you are feeling and how wonderful it is to have this time to yourself. You can thank yourself for being great, or you can encourage yourself to do something that you have been wanting to do but haven't found the time or confidence to fulfil.

You can make a note to contact a friend and have a good old chat and catch up on all their news . . .

You can write about anything that comes into your mind, so that it is out of your mind and you can drop off into a deep, restful, relaxing, perfect sleep.

Remember to turn the light out . . .

DAY 1

This morning you can wake whenever you wish but please stay in bed until 9.30 a.m. There are several reasons for this.

Being given permission to stay in bed will take away all the worry and sense of guilt about not being up and about doing stuff. Sometimes it is good to make yourself do nothing. We fill our minds with people we must see, jobs we must do, thoughts we must think. We hardly ever say, 'I'm doing nothing this weekend' or 'I'm not going to think about anything for the next few days.' The idea of doing nothing is often seen as bad or negative. To relax your mind, detox yourself of negative thinking, and stop putting pressure on yourself, you are positively expected to lie there and just *do nothing*. Snooze if you insist, drift in and out of sleep if you must, but otherwise *do nothing*.

Lemon juice and hot water

Once it is 9.30 a.m. you can get up. Put on a clean dressing gown or house-coat, go to the kitchen and make yourself a cup of hot water with a good squeeze of lemon juice – quarter of a lemon is enough. Make sure the cup is a large one, as this will help towards your daily target of 1.5 litres (3 pints) of water. Starting the day with a squeeze of fresh lemon juice in a cup of hot water will clean your palate and help to flush out your liver (the main detox organ). The lemon is also alkaline-forming which will help to balance the pH of your body. This is a wonderful way to start the day and an excellent alternative to the stimulant of caffeine in coffee and tea.

Shower to wash away the week

Rinse your hair but do not use shampoo, as your hair will be getting a treatment later in the day.

Water is cleansing and refreshing. Think of all the tension and stress just running off your body and down the plughole. Whilst you are showering or bathing, release any negative thoughts you have in your mind. Just imagine them disappearing down the drain, which is where they belong!

As you finish your shower or bath, turn the water to cold for a few moments. Let the icy cold water run over your entire body for just 30 seconds. Alternatively, when you have finished your bath you can turn on the cold tap as the bath water is draining away, cup your hands under the tap and splash the water all over your body.

This may sound like madness but the combination of hot and cold will increase circulation, tone muscles and reduce muscle tension. It will even make you look younger, due to the tonifying effect. All this for just 30 seconds. If you want more then don't worry, there is a full section on Day 2 of the weekend programme!

Dress comfortably

Pat yourself dry and wrap your hair in a towel. Get dressed in loose, comfortable clothing or pyjamas or your dressing gown or housecoat. Put slippers or socks on. Dry your hair with the towel and comb through with a wide-tooth comb or brush – no need to style it as there is a hair treatment to come later.

Breakfast

You should have bought a good selection of fresh fruit in preparation for your 48-hour detox. Now is the time to pick the fruits you want and prepare them for your breakfast. Fruits contain large amounts of essential vitamins, amino acids, and minerals; they are high in fibre and potassium. They contain very little waste and very few calories. Fruits are nearly entirely goodness. Raw fruit is raw energy, and it cleans the gut very efficiently.

Take time to think exactly:

- Which fruit do you wish to eat?
- How you would like to eat it – sliced, peeled, diced or even with a knife and fork?

- Do you want a smoothie?
- Do you want to juice a selection of fruits?
- Would you like it with herbal tea or just a large cup or mug of warm water?

Rest and relaxation

By now it should be around 10.30 a.m. and after all that activity it's time to relax. Watching TV, reading the newspaper or your company newsletter is not the way to relax – you need some escapism. Detox your day of anything stress-related and spend your time generating normality, peace and tranquillity. You will need a really enjoyable novel or a magazine full of fun articles and frivolous nonsense. Go to your relaxation room and get comfortable, with your feet supported just higher than your hips to help circulation, your back supported with cushions or pillows, and a nice warm blanket or duvet tucked in around you. Spend at least an hour relaxing.

Reflexology treatment

Reflexology is fully explained in the 30-Day Ultimate Detox (see pp. 49–51) but the principles are that our feet are a contact point for the whole body. Meridians, energy channels, nerve endings, and pressure points for every organ or system in the body are found at specific locations in our feet. By working on the feet you can have quite a profound effect on your health, your emotions and your physical condition. According to the principles of reflexology, if there is a block in the flow of energy then the body is thrown out of balance. Working on specific points relating to the problem will remove the blockage and so restore the balance.

Obviously you will not be able to give yourself a professional treatment but by doing a thorough foot massage you will be affecting every part of yourself. Concentrating on areas that feel sore will help to clear blockages and improve the way you feel. Clearing any blockage will also help the body to detox itself.

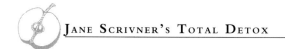

Reflexology massage

To prepare for your home reflexology treatment you will need:

- A bowl for warm water, big enough to put both feet into
- A towel to dry your feet
- Massage oil or calendula powder (optional)
- Pumice or emery board for your feet (optional)

Fill the bowl with warm water and take it to a place where you can sit for 10 minutes soaking your feet. Placing your feet in the warm water will increase the blood flow to them and enhance circulation throughout your body.

When your feet have soaked for 10 minutes you can take them out of the water and dry them off. You might want to use a foot pumice at this stage, to slough away any dead skin on the heels and sides so that you can get to the pressure points more easily.

Now get into a comfortable position, in which you can reach one foot at a time without being too contorted or bent. Follow the sequence as described to rub away the tension and banish the blockages:

- Apply massage oil or powder to your hands (if using).
- Hold your foot with both hands.
- Take a deep breath and using quite firm pressure rub your hands all over your foot and up over your ankle to just below the knee.
- Repeat this stroke three or four times, increasing the pressure as your hands move towards you and decreasing as your hands push away from you.

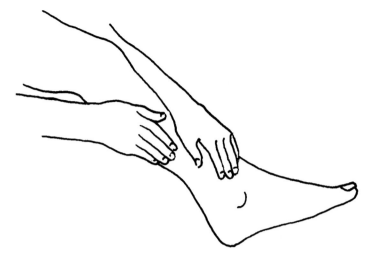

- Place the ends of your fingers together on the sole of your foot with the heels of your hands together on top of your foot.
- Push the heels of your hands out and down, over the top or bridge of your foot, and repeat several times with firm pressure until you have covered the top surface area of your foot.

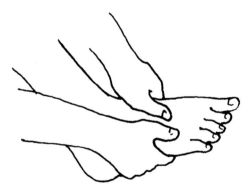

- Leave the heels of your hands together this time and move the ends of your fingers out towards the side of your foot on the underside or sole.
- Rub your foot rigorously.

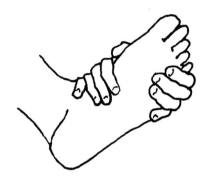

- Place flat hands on the sides of your foot and wiggle it so that all the joints between the toes and foot bones are moved against each other – like you would do to warm up cold feet.

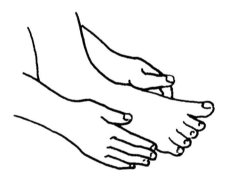

- Using your thumbs, work over the entire surface of your foot in tiny, slow, deep circles. If you are using oil or powder then this stroke works over the skin, as the oil or powder allows 'slipping'. If you are not using oil or powder, the stroke pushes down on the skin and moves it around in small circles.
- Now do the same stroke, working the underside of your foot – remember, lots of very small circles so as not to miss any of the pressure points or reflex points.

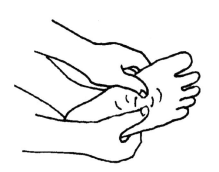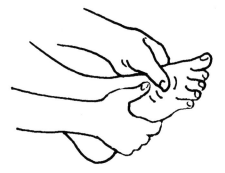

- If you reach an area that is sore you should hold the point with your thumb or finger until the discomfort stops or reduces. Then repeat.
- Squeeze your heel between your thumb and fingers.
- Wiggle each toe along the full length, side and tip. Finish each toe by pulling from the tip with little tugs to open the joints.
- Do some long final strokes all over the foot and up to the knee.
- Once the foot is finished, put on a clean cotton sock. If you used oil don't wash it off, as it will continue to moisturise. Or you can wrap your foot in a towel and then repeat the sequence for your other foot.

Well done! Every last part of you has just had a wonderfully relaxing treatment.

Mid-morning snack

Several small meals are better than two or three big ones so now is the time to have two pieces of fruit and a handful of nuts and/or seeds. You should also take this chance to have a nice cup of hot water – warming, refreshing, cleansing and hydrating for your body and skin.

Yoga stretch session

Yoga and stretching will tone your internal and external organs and muscles. Depending on the types of stretch or yoga you choose, the exercise can be gentle, slow and relaxing or focused and actually quite strenuous.

If you are familiar with stretching exercises, or already attend or have attended a yoga class, then put into practice what you already know. Spend 20 minutes stretching or carrying out your yoga. If not, or if you want to follow instructions so that you do not need to involve your mind in deep thinking at this stage of your detox, then please repeat the following exercise three times.

SUN WORSHIP

Follow the instructions carefully and if at any stage you find the moves difficult or outside your 'stretch range' then just slow down and stay within your comfort zone.

- Stand with your feet shoulder-distance apart, bend your knees slightly and just bounce yourself lightly, rocking from the ball of your feet to the heel, and swinging your arms gently by your side. This will feel as if you are preparing to jump forward from a standing position.

- Breathe deeply through your nose and down into a relaxed belly. Exhale slowly and steadily, and continue to breathe in a relaxed way.

- Bring the palms of your hands together in front of you and lift them slowly until they are directly over your head. If you can, push the stretch slowly until your hands are leaning back past your head. Do not strain anything, just stretch everything.

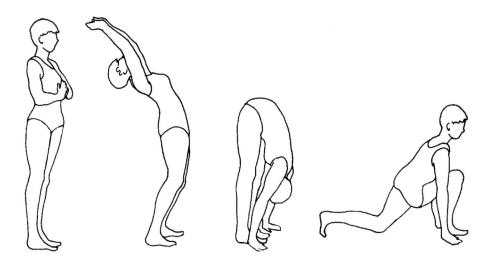

- Now bring your hands forward slowly and roll down to meet your feet, feeling each vertebra stretch as you roll down until your hands touch the floor either side of your feet. Alternatively, just take the stretch to as low as you can manage.

- Let your body flop and your neck relax, with your head hanging down.

- Once in the 'bent double' position, move your left foot back until it is in the biggest stretch behind you with your right foot and both hands in a line on the floor in front of you. This will seem like a lunge and you should feel the stretch in the front of your thigh.

- Now raise your head so that you stretch through your back and neck.

- Lower your head to level with your shoulders, and pull your left foot forward and then your right foot back so that they meet a little past your hips.

- This stretch will feel like a cat stretch. Your back is arched and your head down. Feel the tension in all the muscles as you hold the stretch.

- Lower your body down to touch the floor, you should be lying level with the floor but still supported by your hands and knees.

- Push with your hands to straighten your arms and stretch your stomach muscles, roll your neck and head back as far as you can. Hold the stretch.

- Now do the whole stretch but in reverse, to get back to a relaxed standing position.

- Lower your body flat to the floor.

- Walk your legs up together to the cat stretch, with arched back, hands in front of you and feet behind you.

- Lunge your right foot backwards and leave your right foot between both hands in a line in front of you.

- Pull your right leg up into line with your left leg and stretch into the bent double position.

- Roll your spine up slowly to lift your arms up over your head and past your shoulders.

- Bring your arms back to above your head and then lower them
  to the front of your chest, palms together.

- Take a deep breath and repeat twice more.

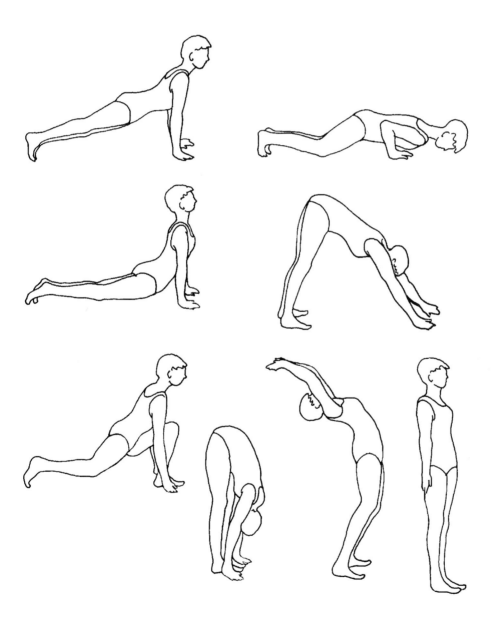

This stretch will move through each and every part of your body from head to toe. It will expand your lungs and deepen your breathing, and will calm and relax you as you salute the sun.

Relaxation lounge

Retire to your quiet room and do some reading for 15 minutes before lunch – you deserve it.

Lunch

Detox food can be wonderfully exotic and yet very basic. Fresh, raw or lightly cooked ingredients will feed your body energy and goodness. Keeping the foods we eat pure and fresh means that we get maximum nutrients for energy and growth. Whereas eating additives, preservatives and toxic chemicals means we use our energy to process what we eat and get rid of most of it – probably with no nutritional gain at all.

You can make any recipe using foods from the lists in the User's Manual but here is a suggested menu:

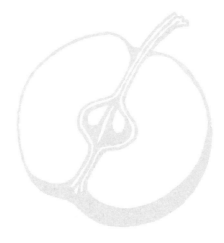

Grilled Fish or Goat's Cheese Salad

Grilled fish or goat's cheese roulade
Fragrant brown rice
Freshly tossed green salad

Boil the short-grain brown rice in the water with a stick of lemongrass and a couple of lime leaves; the flavour will be absorbed by the rice as it cooks. Brown rice usually takes about 30 minutes to cook through so do this first.

If you are having the fish option, choose a piece of fish. Any cut is fine and oily fish is best. Grill until cooked through and the skin is nice and crispy – usually just a few minutes each side.

If you are having the goat's cheese roulade, take some soft goat's cheese, and finely chop some coriander and fresh parsley or any thin-leaved herb of your choice. If the cheese you choose has a rind around it, simply press the soft sides of the cheese into the herb mix, flip over and do the same on the other side. If you wish, place the cheese on a plate and lightly grill until the top of the cheese is melted. If you are using a very soft 'creamy' goat's cheese, just stir in the herbs and shape into a round pattie.

For the salad, place any green leaves (e.g. rocket, lettuce, watercress, mustard, cress, spring onions, Chinese leaf) in a bowl and drizzle with some olive oil. Take half a lemon and half a lime and squeeze the juice of both onto the salad. Toss until the salad is coated with the dressing.

To serve, place a large tablespoon of brown rice on the salad and mix around. Use more rice if you wish, and then transfer the mixture onto your plate and spread so that it covers the entire plate.

Place either the grilled fish or cheese roulade on the top and garnish with some flatleaf parsley and/or coriander.

Now, eat your lunch nice and slowly. Savour every mouthful and see if you can detect all the wonderful flavours, the herbs, the fish or cheese, the salad, the oil and citrus juice . . . And remember, it takes 20 minutes for your stomach to tell your brain that it is full, so take it nice and slow to make sure you don't over-eat.

Country walk to indulge the senses

Now it's time to get some fresh air – one of the best ways to blow away the cobwebs. Taking a walk gives you time to actually see what is going on all around you. We spend so much time 'doing' that we rarely take time to 'be'. Whatever is going on, good or bad, easy or difficult, the flowers still grow, the wind still blows, the sun comes up, the moon comes out, the rain falls and feeds the earth, the clouds scud across the sky, night falls, the stars come out and then day breaks. There is nothing we can do, nothing we can say, nothing we *need* to do and nothing we *have* to say, to make any of it happen. Nature is a constant and as such it is reliable, a place of refuge. Even in the bleakest weather or the wildest storms it just happens and goes on happening. Nature is actually amazing but we never stop to see it, to drink in the changes and the constants. Earth, water, air, fire and metal are all completely natural and from the earth. Everything we do in life comes from these natural elements but we don't pay any attention to it.

After lunch you *can* pay some attention to it. Go for a walk. If it is cold then wrap up warm and if it is hot then make sure you have protection from the sun. Go for a walk and just be with nature. Hug a tree – see what it is that people joke about and see how it feels. Stop and actually look at a flower, its petals, its centre, its stem. Actually smell the fragrance. Don't just think that you know it smells nice – take the time to bend down or reach up and smell the perfume for yourself. Think how wonderful it is that nature makes things smell so nice. I could go on for days about how we should be with nature more, how it can balance and restore. But it won't take you long to discover this for yourself if you just take this time to go out and about and see, feel, touch and smell.

Meditation

Once back from your walk, come inside to the warm, sit quietly and meditate. Meditation releases tension, relaxes our systems and muscles and slows down the frantic brain activity which we seem to live by. Meditation makes you focus on what is now, on what is happening in this moment. Everything that has gone before and everything to come is irrelevant and should be ignored. Meditation is about being in the moment. Relax and concentrate on now.

MEDITATION

You will have already done the following in order to do your Weekend Detox but just make sure:

- Your room is warm and quiet.
- Everyone is out and no one is due to call.
- You have put the ansaphone on or unplugged the phone.

Choose a position that you can stay in for 20 minutes without any discomfort.

For instance:

- You can lie on your back, with your legs and lower back supported by a cushion. Arms should be by your side with palms facing upwards.
- You may decide to sit cross-legged and this is sometimes helped by placing a cushion under your buttocks so that your pelvis is slightly tilted forwards and your back kept straight.

- You may sit upright with your feet placed sole to sole and your knees simply relaxed and resting on the floor.

Now decide on your mantra or chant. A mantra can be a saying, a thought or a wish. For instance:

I am happy, I am healthy, I am peaceful, I am calm
I am happy, I am healthy, I am peaceful, I am calm . . .

You could start by simply saying your own name in a slow rhythm, or just hum the word 'Om' to yourself. Whatever you choose should be low and rhythmic, as it works best if the sound resonates through your muscles as you repeat it.

You should concentrate mainly on your mantra/chant and your breathing. Start with some deep breathing. Breathing correctly will help you through every situation you face, and will greatly enhance your meditation. Deep breathing can calm and soothe, it can help you gather your thoughts, and it can give you balance and concentration. (For a complete relaxation and deep breathing sequence, see the User's Manual, pp.170–3.)

Your meditation should only take 20 or 30 minutes. Get comfortable and get into *you*. Detox those worries about things that may never happen and pass over the things that have gone before. The only thing that is truly real is the moment you are in.

Head wrap and scalp massage

Having a 'bad hair day' can make even the most resilient person feel drab and dull. Our hair is such an important part of the way we look and feel. The first thing most of us do in a time of crisis is to have a totally different haircut or colour – 'I just felt like a change.' It seems to mark a new start.

So, now is the time to boost your crowning glory. Obviously the best way to maintain a shining head of healthy hair is to make sure that your diet is balanced and full of fresh fruit and vegetables. But there are some further measures you can take to ensure glossy, healthy hair.

SCALP MASSAGE

- First you need to get a large towel that can easily be wrapped around your head and secured for 15–20 minutes. Using a small one will result in some of the mixture dribbling out and onto your face which is definitely not conducive to relaxation!

- Take a large ripe avocado, 3 tablespoons of extra-virgin olive oil and a tablespoon of clear honey. Mash the ingredients together until you have a delicious-looking, green paste. Put to one side – in the fridge if possible.

- Now take a cup of natural apple juice and get into position over a sink or bath. Slowly drizzle the juice into your hair until it is completely soaked through to the scalp.

- Still leaning over the sink/bowl/bath, place both hands on your scalp either side of your head (as if you are blocking your ears). Lift your hands off your scalp, leaving only the tips of your fingers in touch with your head and push firmly into the flesh. Massage firmly, pushing the skin across the surface of the skull and not working through your actual hair. (You need to stimulate the deeper muscles so you need to push firmly and slowly in small circles.) Once you have worked an area, you can move the ends of your fingers slightly and start the process again until you have covered your whole head. Move rhythmically and slowly and keep your shoulders relaxed.

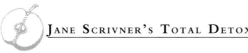

- Now release the skin from your fingertips, grab large clumps of hair in your fists and move these in slow relaxing circles. Pull and tug the hair gently to help increase the blood flow to the roots of the hair.

- Lift your fingers onto your scalp and then tap the ends of all your fingers in a brisk movement onto your scalp. This should feel like a tapping movement across the entire surface of your head.

- Relax. Take the avocado blend from where you have stored it and work it into the roots of your hair. Lift your hair in sections and cover the roots in the mixture. Once all the roots are covered, start to coat all the remaining hair. When you have covered all your hair, smooth it around your head and pull into a little point on top. (This part is optional but it is exactly what you did in the bath aged four, when your head was covered in shampoo!) Wrap your entire head in the towel and relax for 15–20 minutes. Let the heat of your head 'cook' your hair.

- When the time is up, remove the towel and rinse your hair in hand-hot water. Make sure you rinse absolutely all the mixture off and then lightly shampoo your hair. Towel-dry your hair and let it dry naturally – no need to use heated rollers or a blow-drier as you are just 'at home' this evening.

Relaxation session

You now have time to relax totally. Choose a favourite film, curl up with a book or simply snooze. Make sure you keep warm, especially if your hair is still damp. Don't feel guilty about doing nothing. Positively *expect* to do nothing and enjoy every minute of it. Each time a thought enters your head that is not to do with how you are relaxing right now, just let it pass right through. Concentrate on how you are feeling, how relaxed your scalp is, how good the book is, how enjoyable the film is, how cosy you feel, how wonderful it is to just relax and re-energise – feel good right now.

Suppertime

You should now be ready to glide into the kitchen and prepare a delicious supper. Make sure you lay the table and have a comfortable seat. You should also try to eat by 6.30 p.m. as this is the last meal you will have before commencing your secret mini fast (see the User's Manual, p. 190).

Chew each mouthful before taking the next one, and put your knife and fork down between each mouthful. See if you can actually taste everything you have prepared, instead of finishing the meal without having even registered what you have cooked.

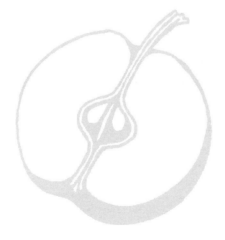

Thai vegetable soup with a spicy vegetable grill

For the Thai vegetable soup, you need:

A selection of vegetables (e.g. carrots, courgettes, red onions,
    any variety of squash, green beans)
1 vegetable stock cube, crumbled
1 stick of lemongrass
1 chilli, halved
Some goat's or sheep's yoghurt
Fresh coriander

Chop all the vegetables, place them in a pan and just cover with water. Bring to the boil with the stock cube, lemongrass and chilli. Mix thoroughly together. When the vegetables are tender remove the pan from the heat and drain the stock into a bowl. Remove the chilli and lemongrass and blend the vegetables together. Add the stock and yoghurt to get a soup-like consistency. When your spicy vegetables are ready, serve with the soup sprinkled with the chopped coriander.

For the spicy vegetable grill, you need:

A large portion of mixed vegetables (courgettes, red and white
    onions, broccoli, potatoes, fennel)
1 small beetroot
1 teaspoon freshly grated ginger root
Some crumbled goat's cheese

Preheat the oven to 180°C/350°F/Gas Mark 4. Slice the vegetables into thin strips. Place them in a large preheated, ovenproof dish, stir in the crushed ginger and sprinkle the goat's cheese on top. Bake in the oven for 40 minutes until the vegetables are tender and the goat's cheese nicely browned.

Dry float relax

Obviously you cannot lie down and relax immediately after you have eaten. Once you feel ready, you can create your own 'dry float'. Place all the cushions from the sofa on the floor and have enough cushions around to support the back of your legs, head and arms – have a cushion to support your lower back if you need it. Place candles on tables and mantelpieces – anywhere safe where there can be no risk of them catching fire or falling over while you have your eyes closed.

Play some relaxing music of your choice and start to get into position. Lay all the cushions on the floor, and place a pillow underneath your thighs to keep your back flat on the floor. Place a cushion underneath your ankles so that your feet are supported. Put a nice soft pillow under your head and neck and, if you have enough left, place a pillow under each arm. You should feel totally supported, with your limbs slightly higher than your torso – as if you are floating in water. Take some deep breaths and listen to the relaxing music. Stay just where you are for at least 30 minutes . . . mmmmmmmmmmmmmmmm.

Natural manicure and hand massage

You may wish to do this treatment sitting up in bed, as it's best to keep your hands wrapped and warm for as long as possible after the treatment. Overnight would be fabulous – your hands will emerge moisturised and refreshed the following day. So, take yourself off, clean your teeth and get into bed. This massage is really quite simple but a wonderful way to scrub away all the dry, dead skin from your hands, to moisturise deeply and to increase the circulation to the 'tools' that we use all day every day but never give a second thought to.

Hand massage

You will need:

- Some natural sea salt
- A few drops of lavender essential oil
- Some olive oil
- Some cotton gloves (if you cannot get hold of cotton gloves then use hand towels or towelling/flannel mitts)

Mix 1 tablespoon of natural sea salt with ½ tablespoon of olive oil and 3–4 drops of essential oil.

Scoop the scrub mix onto each hand and rub your hands together, slowly at first, building up to a firm 'wringing' motion. Make sure you cover the entire hand and wrist area and rub together for a couple of minutes. Leave for 1 minute, then rinse your hands gently in warm water.

There may be a slightly oily residue but this is fine. Dip your hands in a little more olive oil and then begin to massage:

- Wring your hands as if really washing them thoroughly.

- Lean your thumb into the wrist area of the other hand and, in small firm circles, move over the entire area of your wrist and the top of your hand.

- Place the heel of one hand over the top of the other hand and open out across the top of the hand.

- Lean your thumb down between each bone on one hand and drain towards the wrist.

- Lean your thumb into the back of one hand and move the flesh across the bones in a circular motion.

- Turn the hand over slowly and lean your thumb into the palm. Move over the entire palm in small firm circles in an up and outwards motion, paying special attention to the ball of the hand.

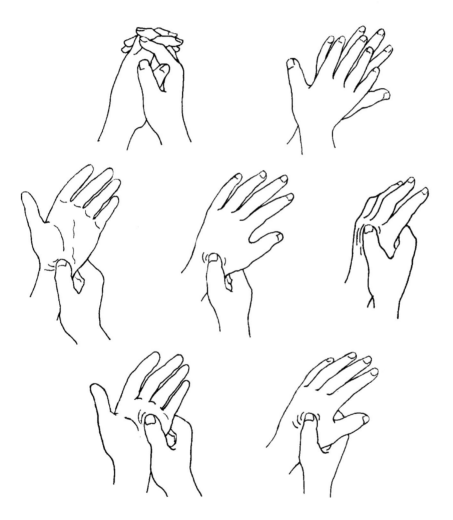

- Now repeat the whole sequence with the other hand.

- Squeeze, wring and stretch fingers individually.

- Push back the cuticles slowly and firmly, using the side of your thumbs. Do not use another nail as this may tear the cuticle.

- Rub your hands together for one last time. Then put on the cotton gloves or wrap your hands in the towels or mitts.

Snuggle down, turn off the lights and sleep like a baby.

DAY 2

Awake slowly and get up. Remove your oily towels or mitts and place in the laundry basket.

Dress slowly and warmly in preparation for your early morning walk.

As you did yesterday, start the day with hot water and lemon juice (see p. 99). Be sure not to eat anything, as you are now well into your mini fast.

A refreshing walk

Take a refreshing walk – nothing too brisk, as you are likely to be feeling hungry. Remember the walk you took yesterday and take the time to have a look at what is growing and what is changing.

Stretch and relax

Follow the stretches from yesterday to waken and salute the sun (see p. 106). Feel your body and lungs expand, taking in refreshing air and exhaling any stale, used air.

Exfoliating scrub, thermotherapy bath and body drench

Now it's time to treat yourself to a full body purge. You will totally exfoliate, take a relaxing and invigorating bath, and finish with a refreshing moisture drench.

Sloughing off dead skin cells helps circulation and allows the skin to breathe more efficiently, which in turn prepares you for the therm-otherapy bath. The combination of hot and cold has been used for hundreds of years in such treatments. The Kneipp school in Germany has long promoted the use of hot and cold baths to stimulate circulation and natural healing. Spas have existed for just as long, with people in Scandinavia and others countries bathing in varying degrees of hot, warm, cool and cold waters. Closing with an application of a simple moisture lotion all over will complete your detox experience.

Be prepared to feel a little tired and keep your fluid intake up, as anything that increases circulation will also increase the need for water. And anything involving heat will require your water levels to be maintained.

HOME SPA

Ideally you should have access to a bath *and* shower. If not, then a bath with a shower head or just a shower will do; you need to be able to access lots of hot and cold water in very quick succession.

- Begin by closing all the windows in your bathroom and putting a large bath mat on the floor. Turn the radiator up to full to get the heat really high.

- Run a hot bath, allowing the steam to build up in the room. Stay in the room while the bath is running and benefit from the steam opening your pores and your body beginning to sweat.

- Mix together a handful of natural sea salt, a cup of olive oil and a few drops of peppermint essential oil.

- Standing on a mat or towel, rub the mixture all over your entire body, rubbing firmly to slough off any dead or dry skin.

- Once you have thoroughly exfoliated, stand in a warm shower and continue to rub the salt mix until it has all rinsed away. You should feel invigorated and your skin will have a nice tingle.

- Get in the bath and relax for 10 minutes.

- When your 10 minutes is up, get out of the bath and turn on the shower or turn the shower head to cold. Stand under the cold water for a count of 20 seconds. If you only have a shower attachment for your bath then just cool your head, arms and upper body over the sink.

- Jump back into the hot bath and relax for just 5 minutes.

- Get back under the shower for a count of 20 seconds.

- Get back into the bath for 5 minutes.

- Finish with a cold shower for just 10 seconds.

- Wrap yourself in a warm towel and relax for 5 minutes.

- Remove the towel and, whilst the bathroom is still warm, apply the moisturiser of your choice all over your body. Rub it in and don't be mean. You need to drench your body in moisture, inside and out: total rehydration.

Relaxation session

You won't need to be talked into this session; you are probably feeling relaxed and nicely tired. You have not had anything to eat today so please make sure you have some water or herbal tea. Go to your chosen relaxation place and make sure your feet are wedged up with pillows or cushions until they are higher than your hips. This will help the lymph to flow whilst you are sitting still. (It is normally pumped around the body as you move your muscles, but putting your feet up enables gravity to do the job just as well.)

Light lunch of tisanes and assorted grapes

During this mini fast you are allowing your body to rest and cleanse. By taking it easy physically, you are giving your muscles and internal organs a break as well.

Settle down to a large bunch of grapes and a cup of warm water with a peppermint leaf in it, or a cup of peppermint tea.

Eat slowly, crushing the grapes on the roof of your mouth with your tongue or between your teeth. Feel the juice, full of goodness, flood your mouth – cleansing, refreshing and revitalising.

Relaxation, reading, journal writing or just drifting

After lunch you will want to rest. This can take any form you wish but certainly you should get yourself into a comfortable, supported position and keep warm. You can take this time to read a good book, write your thoughts in a diary or just to sit and contemplate anything that comes to mind. The subject must be you: how you are, how you feel and how you are thinking. Take this time to indulge yourself. Don't think about anything relating to work or family or other obligations. You deserve some special thought. You may even drift off and dream, but make sure you dream about *you*!

List writing and right-drawer compilation

When you have relaxed and woken, write down some thoughts about what you want in your life, what your plans are for the future and what your plans are for the present. You have remained in the present up to this stage of your 48-hour detox but now you can allow yourself to move to the future.

Writing things down serves many purposes:

- It gets them out of your mind and so clears the clutter.
- It means they are written visually, so you can look at your thoughts, wishes and ideas and not just think them. This gives you a new perspective.
- It preserves your thoughts so that you don't waste time trying to remember them.
- It means you think them through differently as you write them.
- It means you can revisit them and think new thoughts about them without confusion.
- It means you can tick them off, as you do them, as they come true, and as they are no longer relevant.
- It detoxes your mind, freeing you up for clearer thoughts and bigger plans and dreams.

I also once heard that if you write something down that is troubling you, or that you really want, and place it in your right-hand drawer – wherever that may be – then eventually it will come true, come right or just go away, whatever would be the best solution. This introduces the power of positive thought and putting things out for the universe to deal with. It does not mean abdicating responsibility but it does mean being open to any help there is on offer. Try it and see what happens – it might just work.

CANDLE MEDITATION

Well done, you are nearing the end of your mini fast and your 48-hour Weekend Detox. You should be feeling well and truly refreshed and cleansed. Before allowing yourself time to prepare for your guests this evening, you can finish with a candle mediation.

Light a candle and place it so that the flame is about eye level when you are sitting comfortably. Cross your legs, keep your back straight, turn your palms to face the ceiling and rest the back of your hands on your thighs. Breathe deeply into your stomach and relax (see User's Manual, pp. 170–2).

- Concentrate on the flame and its glow of energy. Watch the light move and flicker but burn on.

- Watch how any small draught can all but put out the flame. Then watch it come back and burn just as brightly and intensely.

- See how the flame moves as you exhale slowly and steadily through your open mouth.

- Imagine you are breathing the warmth of the flame into your belly as you inhale.

- See the golden light and imagine it travelling through your body with every breath. Let it replace the dull and lifeless breath you exhale until you are totally filled with warm golden light.

- Close your eyes and see the flame as your focus. Stay there for a few moments.

- Slowly open your eyes and unfold your legs.

- Push yourself up to a standing position and then shake all your limbs loose.

- Take one last deep breath, do a full stretch so that your arms are extended over your head, hold it and relax.

Well done . . . you are totally detoxed.

Light supper

Now all you need to do is prepare a lovely meal to share with your friends/partner or family. Make sure you eat after 6.30 p.m. to truly complete your mini fast but prepare any foods of your choice from the lists in the User's Manual (see pp. 160–3). Make sure it's something light. Grilled fish and salad, followed by fresh fruit for dessert, would be good choices.

Don't stay up too late. You should be in bed by 10.30 p.m. but listen to your own body. If you feel tired before this then bid your friends a good evening, thank them for coming and take yourself off to bed.

Morning 3

Having finished your programme and had a nourishing night's sleep, you should start the day with a wonderful nut crunch muesli or fresh fruit muesli – whichever you prefer.

Whilst sipping a cup of hot water and lemon, mix together the seeds, nuts and/or fruit (fresh or dried) with natural goat's or sheep's yoghurt and tuck in. Chew slowly and taste the raw energy. What a great way to start the day.

Once again, well done and good luck! You never know what may lie in store for the new, refreshed, cleansed and detoxed you . . .

5 The Complete Home Detox

Our **homes are one of** the most important things in our lives. We put so much effort and money, so many desires, hopes and dreams into them. So why not look at ways to make our homes perfect for us and the people we share them with?

Detoxing your home means getting rid of everything and anything that could bring negative energy, destructive influence or just a bad vibe. In this programme you will find ways to make every room feel happy, comforting, energising and relaxing. You will also find ways to make your life, and the lives of those around you, more prosperous and successful, more enriched and more valued.

Families, relationships and jobs are all hugely important of course but if you do not have a real home to go to, to find comfort in, to protect you, or just to spend time in, then it is difficult to find happiness in these other areas.

Our homes are one of the biggest expenses in our lives. However we live – owner occupier, rental, lodgings, hotel, houseboat, council house, private island! – we have either paid a huge sum upfront or we pay a substantial monthly fee. If you own your home you are likely to have paid somewhere between £40,000 and £400,000 – whichever it is you probably only saw the place two or three times before signing on the dotted line. What an amazing leap of faith! And what better reason to ensure that you make the most of your investment?

Do you need to detox your home?

If you answer yes to any of the following – not just at home but in any part of your life – then detoxing your home is just what you need to do. Some may seem obvious and some quite strange but all can be helped, improved or eradicated by at least one of the detox tools this book describes:

- Do you feel drained at home?
- Do you have a room that seems too dark?
- Do you often suffer from health problems?
- Do you suffer sleepless nights?
- Are you unsuccessful in relationships?
- Do you feel confused or unsettled?
- Are you trying for children?
- Do you have recurrent nightmares?
- Do you want to be more successful in your job?
- Do you want to earn more money?
- Do you want to feel happier?
- Do you want more energy?
- Could you do with more time?
- Do you sense that you have ghosts?
- Do you feel something is not right?
- Do you have an unfriendly house?

- Were the last people to live in your home unhappy or ill or divorcing?
- Do you want to move but feel unable to get away?
- Do you need change but just cannot make the break?
- Could you have more relaxation in your life?
- Do you need more space?
- Do unwelcome people keep coming into your home?
- Are there things that are broken or need fixing in your home?
- Would you like to improve the quality of your life?

Do any of these problems sound familiar? If so, read on . . .

What do you need to do?

Follow the five-point plan to change the way you live and add some colour and sparkle to your home and surroundings. In order to detox your home you need to open your mind to everything that you wish to change and improve in your life. You must also look at your home and see what you truly want to change or improve, and also register areas that just don't feel right though you can't put your finger on why. Consider areas that shouldn't be the way they are, or that were not right when you moved in. Consider anything that may be causing you problems because the Complete Home Detox can almost certainly do something about it.

> Feng Shui the fug and space-clear the clutter, or simply spring-clean the cupboards.

Give your home a makeover and feel the benefit of getting things in the right place and looking after your home. Welcome the ghosts and banish the bad vibes – live in peace and harmony and let your surroundings work for you.

The Complete Home Detox can also work at work. Try the plan with your colleagues or friends and see just how good it feels to get things sorted.

THE FIVE-POINT PLAN

1: Get rid of clutter and apply the six-month rule
2: Now is the time to spring-clean
3: Detox your space
4: Banish electromagnetic fields
5: Get support from your surroundings

1: Get rid of clutter and apply the six-month rule

In order to completely detox your home you need to assess and prioritise and then expel all the waste and 'stuff'. Old clothes, furniture, goods and kitchen items count as 'stuff'. Go through all your posessions and sort them into piles of things you definitely want, piles of things you don't want, and then things you are not sure about. Enliven your environment, detox unwanted clutter, invigorate your energies and forge your way forward. Removing everything that gets in the way, or is not beautiful or useful, gives you a clean fresh approach to life.

Your home is full of furniture, books, records, contents of old Christmas crackers, buttons that don't match, single socks, old school textbooks, broken bits, clothes, shoes, hats and scarves that have been part of your life for a long time. We buy new stuff to replace out-of-date or worn-out stuff that we hardly ever throw out or give away.

Now is the time to bag up all the things you don't want and take them to a clothing agency or charity shop or donate them to a jumble sale that will benefit some local cause – or even experience the joys of the car boot sale. Keep what you want and put them back in their drawers or cup-boards. You should, by now, have lots more space. Place all the things you are not sure about in a bag, store them somewhere out of the way and apply the six-month rule – if you don't use the contents for six months then take them all to the local charity shop, dress agency or jumble sale. Many other people can benefit from your own detoxing and you will benefit because you have removed all the stale unwanted goods from your home.

Detoxing your office will help you clear your mind to make the energy flow and your business grow and prosper! You need to go through the same process as detoxing your home but in your own office environment. Go through all your files and see if anything has been duplicated or is no longer relevant. You need to make your own decision, depending on the type of business, as to how much filing must be kept as current. For instance you could set up 'archive files' so that day-to-day paperwork is easier to access.

You may want to start by simply 'putting your affairs in order'. Instigate a filing system if you don't already have one. Put invoices in date order. Find a place for an efficient petty cash record. Label files so that you do not need to open them and trawl through them just to find out their contents.

Feng Shui your desk by clearing away all the clutter from the surface. If you have a messy desk then you will have a messy business. And if you cannot see the work space in front of you for piles of papers then you cannot have a clear route forward for your business.

Have your workplace or desk facing into a room and not directly facing a wall. Again, the rules of Feng Shui state that facing a wall means that you have no view of the future and your progress is blocked.

Detox your handbag or your briefcase – even the everyday things that you use without any thought can be detoxed. For instance, look through your briefcase and remove all the old receipts, old documents, and pens that don't work (and carry a pen that actually does). Put all the small change swilling about in the bottom of your bag into a pot, together with all the change from down the side of your sofa. It may even add up to the price of a pint or a glass of wine every now and then! Try carrying one or two lipsticks that have colour left in them instead of a selection of old fluffy ones that have snapped off and you don't wear anyway. Take a look at your personal organiser. Are you still carrying last year's diary pages? They could be filed safely at home and save you the trouble of flicking to the wrong year every time you try to fix a meeting.

Even small things, like keyrings, can be detoxed. I recently went through mine and realised that I had had keys cut to give to three people, moved offices before handing them out, and was still carrying three out-side door keys to a building I didn't work in and which had changed its locks anyway.

Remember, if there is any doubt as to whether you need something, simply bag it up and store it for six months; if you don't give it a second thought then you obviously don't need it any more and someone else can probably benefit from it. Take the bag to the local charity shop and feel good about yourself and your newly detoxed home.

2: Now is the time to spring-clean

Once you have rid yourself of all the things you don't want or need then you can clean and I really mean clean – a good old-fashioned roll-your-sleeves-up spring-clean.

A complete spring-clean will take a good long time. Depending on the size of the house or rooms, it could even take several days. It means opening every drawer, every cupboard and every shelf and cleaning. Not tidying but cleaning. You should have tidied away all your unwanted poses-sions and rubbish by now, but if you haven't then you must do this *before* attempting a full spring-clean. If you don't tidy up first you may well find that you spend time cleaning something you then give or throw away. Point 2 must always follow point 1!

Take a long look at the size of your project and work out how long you want to spend on the job. There is no rule that says you have to do the whole task in one go. You may decide to do one room per week, you may decide to do three hours per evening until the job is complete, but whatever you decide try to stick to it. This will ensure that your five-point plan will be completed before it is time to start all over again. If you have a very messy family you may find that unless you do the whole project in a relatively short period of time, they will make sure you cannot tell exactly where you have cleaned from where you haven't reached yet! Choose your time and go for it.

Spring-cleaning activities

Here's a check list of tasks:

- Empty cupboards
- Wipe shelves
- Wipe jars and lids
- Vacuum under furniture
- Dust tops of cupboards and wardrobes
- Clean walls
- Clean fingerprints off doors
- Wipe marks off windows
- Clean mirrors
- Shake rugs
- Wash sheets
- Take winter coats to dry-cleaners to pack away for the winter or wash summer clothes and put away for next summer

- Clean the stair rods
- Polish the brass
- Wipe the door knobs
- Polish the floors
- Rinse the soap dishes
- Wipe the shower cubicle
- Wash the bath
- Clean the toothpaste dribbles
- Wash the net curtains or wipe the blinds
- Dry-clean the curtains and upholstery
- Beat the mats

Go behind everything, on top of everything, around everything and under everything . . . In short, do whatever is required to get absolutely everything clean.

Play music loudly, sing and boogie around the house and just think of all the dirt, dust, grime and rubbish you are detoxing from your life – and that's just the clean houses!

3: Detox your space

Once you have spring-cleaned your space it is time to 'clear' it. Space clearing is the art of cleansing and consecrating buildings and homes. This works on two levels – physical and spiritual.

The physical removal of rubbish, dirt and clutter   The most common culprits are: old magazines and newspapers, old clothes that you no longer wear, old foods that are past their sell-by date, crockery you don't use, old saucepans that have been replaced by newer cleaner varieties, old make-up you never wear, old medicines you never finished and should have thrown away for safety's sake, old bubble baths that have never been used, the contents of several years of Christmas crackers that you cannot bear to throw away . . . Need I say more, except that applying the six-month rule from point 1 and spring-cleaning in point 2 will sort this out for sure.

The spiritual removal of stale, stagnant, negative energy or actual removal or recognition of energetic entities (ghosts)   Rooms you don't use, photo albums you have never sorted, thoughts you have never told your loved ones, apologies that have gone unheard, confessions not made, arguments left unsettled . . .

For the purposes of the Complete Home Detox we are going to look at simple space clearing techniques for you to start to introduce at home. There are many practitioners who would be more than happy to come to your home or office and space-clear for you. But it might be good to start by seeing just what sort of difference you can make by introducing a few simple techniques.

At its most elementary level, space clearing is just like physical spring-cleaning. On a deeper level it is about actually cleaning the energy of your home and thus renewing it and making it fully active.

How to start   You should start by realising that you will not be able to take on the whole house overnight! Clearing should be done thoroughly and systematically – the process should be as ordered and energetic as you wish your home to be once you have completed your clearing.

Choose the room you spend most time in and then you should feel the benefits of your clearing much quicker. Once you have chosen your room – perhaps your living room – begin. It will be easy to see all the items that can be discarded almost immediately: rubbish, out-of-date magazines, old wrappers, the contents of the rubbish bin (if you haven't done this already). There is nothing scientific about throwing away all the rubbish. The next step is to look at all the items in the room and decide if you really need or want them in there. This is not to say that you should leave your room as empty as possible. You may like a lot of furniture. You just need to make sure that you are only left with useful, practical or beautiful items.

Once the room is clear of waste, you need to set about physically cleaning it. Move all the furniture, vacuum behind everything and clean away the stale dust that has settled behind the sofa or taken up residence behind the Rembrandt! Polish any surfaces and wipe any windows. Clean the telephone receiver and remove any dead leaves or flowers from house plants. Check down the side of the chairs for crumbs or coins and shake up the cushions into full 'plump'.

> Ensure that the room is exactly how you would want it to be if you were arriving home after a long hard day, ready to make you feel welcome and relaxed.

You can then go on to do every room in the house in the same way, following the steps below.

Note

Space clearing will not be understood by everyone. So if you decide to space-clear your own home it's best to do it alone when everyone else is out. To encourage the flow and cleansing of energy within your home you should nurture it. We talk to friends, pets and even plants. Now it's time to talk to your home.

- Wear loose comfortable clothing and relax into your task. You need to be receptive to the 'vibe' you get back from your rooms.

- You can use chimes and bells to clear space, you can use aromatherapy essential oils and you can use flowers and petals. If the weather is fine you should open the windows and let the air flow, and you can use incense or candles to encourage energy to circulate.

- Wander round the room and feel each and every part of it. Identify areas that feel colder and flatter and areas that feel energetic and active. Go around clapping loudly into each and every area to chase out the stagnant energy and move around the active energy. Clap low and high.

- Scatter petals or spray essential oils in a water solution lightly around the room. Use a chime to sound in the darkest corners and highest points and move the energy around every nook and cranny. Light candles to draw the air and circulate the atmosphere.

- Before you finish, walk around the perimeter of the room and stroke the energy in, encouraging forward motion – as if encouraging something to pass you by. Once you have done this, the energy should be evenly distributed, cleansed and refreshed.

- Clear away your cleansing equipment. Then see how the room feels and how you feel about what you have just achieved.

Search where you wish – not a jot of tox will be found, physically, emotionally or spiritually.

4: Banish electromagnetic fields

Detox electronic, magnetic, microwave, metallic and ozone stress from your life and live 'charge free'. Now that your home is detoxed, your rooms are clean and your space is cleared, you can vanquish the negative vibes.

The influence of technology on our lives is incredibly liberating. We can get in touch with people via mobile phones wherever they are; we can microwave our food in a fraction of the time it takes to cook conventionally. The television brings us all the news and entertainment for a fun-packed evening and when we turn in for the night we can snuggle into the warmth of a heated electric blanket. We are woken on request by our radio alarm chirping at our bedside and we shower and then style our hair using electric dryers and heated curling tongs.

Life could hardly be more convenient but all this convenience comes at a cost. The increase in electromagnetic fields (EMFs) is partly to blame. We already have natural electromagnetic radiation from the sun and earth but reports say that we are now bombarded with 150 million times more electromagnetic signals than our grandparents were.

You only need to drive under an electricity pylon and hear the radio frequency fuzz to experience the effect of an electromagnetic field. Likewise, you can turn the radio on near the hairdryer or curling tongs and you will also get interference. Listen to a battery-operated radio and hear the buzz when the washing machine does its spin cycle two floors away. These are all examples of electromagnetic radiation travelling through our day-to-day lives and our bodies.

But is this really bad for us or is it just another media-hyped health scare? Research suggests that it *is* bad, and it could well be a cause of many, many illnesses, diagnosed or otherwise. Roger Coghill is a leading expert in electropollution and lectures frequently on the subject. His view is that our bodies have their own electrical frequencies, involved in growth, repair and cellular renewal; and that electric fields from machines and mobiles, microwaves and so on all have a detrimental effect on these personal frequencies. According to his research, it is the alternating current (or AC) part of the electromagnetic field that is dangerous to us, and this exists all the time when an appliance is plugged in or fully charged.

It is suggested that illnesses such as ME, lethargy, headaches and some cancers are the result of our bodies' inability to repel these electric fields. Some people also believe that EMFs disrupt the functioning of our immune systems.

So there are many precautions you can take to reduce all unnecessary exposure to EMFs. Roger Coghill believes we are resilient to short-term exposure; we should simply reduce our constant or longer-term exposure. Even if the final results of the research suggest that there is no real long-term danger or effect we should still do all we can to reduce any potential interference.

How to reduce your EMF exposure

Reports have suggested the following:

- Long-term exposure is most likely to happen whilst you are sleeping in one spot for approximately seven hours per day. For instance, sleeping with a radio alarm can increase your exposure to EMFs at the very time your body needs all its faculties for the job of cell repair (which happens during the sleeping hours). General advice is to move the radio alarm so that it is at least 1.2 metres (4 feet) away. Alternatively, you can resort to the good old-fashioned wind-up alarm clock and get some real rest.

- Electric blankets are reportedly tantamount to actually getting into an electromagnetic field! Even when the blanket is turned off you are still lying on a metallic grid and this will upset your own natural electric fields. Ditch the blanket and just put on a warmer duvet or snuggle up closer.

- Mobile phones are reputed to be causing brain tumours. If you really need to use one, the best advice is to enclose the whole phone in a shield which is available from mobile phone stores.

- Unfortunately our parents were right all along . . . 'Don't sit too close to the television' is an all too familiar phrase from most people's childhood. We've probably used the phrase ourselves to shout at our offspring. Well, research has shown that it's true: we do tend to sit in front of the television for longer periods than any other household item. As they give out negative ions, we should sit no closer than 1.5 metres (5 feet) from the screen.

- Computer screens also give out negative ions. So make sure you work at least 50 centimetres (2 feet) from the screen and take regular breaks. An ioniser can be useful, as it will clear and balance the air of all negativity. They can be bought from major chemists or healthfood shops. You may notice the difference in aches and pains or skin tone in just a few days if you have been working with lots of electronic gadgetry.

- The jury is still out on microwaves, though it's commonly believed that you shouldn't spend too much time close to one once it is turned on and perhaps leave your food for a few minutes before tucking in (a useful piece of advice anyway, as food is generally too hot to eat immediately). You can check the security of your microwave by holding a radio near the door when it is turned on. If there is interference than there is likely to be leakage and repairs must be made or the appliance should be replaced.

Whatever the facts it seems to make sense to reduce the rays.

5: Get support from your surroundings

Having cleared and cleansed your home, you can now move things around to get the best out of what remains.

Why not design our homes so that we bring health, wealth and happiness into our lives as well as patterned borders and bunk beds in the children's room? We spend huge amounts on our houses. And we strive to make the most of our lives by following simple rules of existence that have been passed down from generation to generation. We choose colours we like, we choose houses by the look of them from the driveway, we knock rooms together or extend into open space. We design our gardens for optimum appearance and minimum effort, we search the antique shops for the ultimate doorstop . . .

There are many other cultures that follow their own sets of rules and operate in much the same way. But some of these cultures attach a little more importance to their surroundings than others. In Tibet and Vietnam they follow *Phong Thuy*; in the Philippines, Indonesia and Thailand they follow *Hong Sui*, and in Japan, Hawaii and India they believe in *Vaastu Shastra*.

The Chinese follow the rules and science of Feng Shui (pronounced 'Fung Shway' or 'Fung Shoy'), many of which are being introduced throughout the world due to interest from westerners. Its popularity is partly due to our increasing desire to get the best out of our homes, and more importantly to become happier, healthier and wealthier individuals. Feng Shui supports the desire to make the most of what we have.

According to Derek Walters, who wrote *The Feng Shui Handbook* (published by Thorsons), 'Feng Shui is a philosophy, of Chinese origin, which maintains that the configurations of the earth shape the affairs of the people that live among them.'

The two characters 'Feng' and 'Shui' literally mean 'wind' and 'water'. This really points to the fact that Feng Shui is concerned with earthly rather than spiritual influences. Feng Shui is not a religion or an art; it is a science. It has strict rules and, along with the overall philosophy, it includes many, many tools, techniques and exercises.

To put it simply, Feng Shui is about getting all the positive energy available to you into your life, keeping it there, using it to its optimum, and then allowing all negative energy a free route out of your life. Keeping up a constant flow of good energy, without any blockages, will help bring you health, wealth and prosperity.

There are many schools of Feng Shui and it would be arrogant of me to dictate the school you should follow. But there are many, many books and magazines that you can read to find out the basics.

The best way to ensure that you are following Feng Shui principles is to have a consultation. These can be very expensive but, if you get a fully qualified practitioner who has studied for many years rather than done a few weekend courses (see Useful Addresses), you will find that the results will undoubtedly be worth the initial outlay.

Whilst you are deciding how to introduce Feng Shui into your life, there are some simple steps you can take that will start you on your journey.

As we said earlier, Feng Shui has a lot to do with the flow of energy. For energy to flow all blockages or obstacles need to be removed. Anything that may shut it off or redirect it or prevent it from entering every part of your home should be rectified. In the same way, anything that speeds up the energy too much should also be carefully looked at so that a balanced flow is maintained.

Stand outside your house on the street, face your front door and imagine that you are the positive energy. Look around you and consider whether there is anything that is preventing your easy access to your home.

Is there a tree across your front door? Is your front door old and dirty? Is the drive long and funnel–like so that too much energy speeds up towards the door and overpowers it? Or is the path just long enough for the energy to arrive at the door, ready for entry?

Does the front door work? Does it stick? Get that fixed. Does your hallway lead you through the house? Or is there a wall in the way that blocks the flow? Is there a door you never use or that is blocked by a piece of furniture? If so, clear the blockage and open the door – let the energy flow in.

Have you got mirrors facing each other? As a rule that just bounces energy back and forth, it is disruptive and interferes with the flow. Move the mirrors so that they don't reflect on each other but instead reflect the energy out into the house and encourage its path.

Hang all doors so that they open into the rooms and not back out into the hall or corridor, so that when you approach a room you naturally flow into it. Check that the back door is not blocked and opens outwards. This enables all energy, once it has passed through the house and been used, to exit freely. Check, however, that the front door is not in line with the back door. Otherwise you will find energy entering at the front and then zooming straight out of the back of your property before it gets a chance to circulate its beneficial properties.

Once you have completed your journey through your house you will be more aware of the dynamics of your home and you may wish to make some changes to get the optimum energy flow. You have now completed some basic steps towards implementing Feng Shui into your life. You have detoxed the negative energy and promoted the positive energy. Well done!

6 The Relationship Detox

Partners, friends and family all play an incredibly important part in our lives: sometimes they can make you happy and sometimes they can drive you bananas. You can spend time with someone and feel fabulous or just have a short phone call and want to scream. The Relationship Detox gets you to look at your relationships and see how to get the best out of them, how to boost them and how to know when to leave them alone for a while. Our relationship with ourselves is also incredibly important – until we start treating our self, respecting our self and boosting our self, we cannot expect to be able to do all these things for anyone else. If we are fulfilled than we can give. If we are drained and tired then we need to preserve and boost ourselves back up to full strength. The Relationship Detox will help you look at all areas of your relationships: areas of strength, areas of weakness, areas of opportunity and areas of threat.

WHAT IS A **SWOT** ANALYSIS?

One good way to look at your life is to use a business tool – a SWOT analysis. SWOT stands for Strengths, Weaknesses, Opportunities and Threats; all aspects of your life can be put under one of these four headings. Applying a SWOT analysis can be a very revealing exercise, showing up areas of your life you hadn't even considered worth looking at. It also helps you move forward with some key information about what is useful to you and what is not.

Applying this analysis to any and every part of your life can very quickly bring to light areas that you need to address. You need to be brutally honest! This analysis should also be private and confidential. Whatever your current situation, to truly detox you need to know all the facts. You need to include everything, good or bad, cruel or kind.

A SAMPLE **SWOT** ANALYSIS

This is what a 'Personal SWOT analysis' might look like.

What are your strengths?

These are things that you are good at or that are established and ongoing, things that you are happy with. This list may change but at this moment in time you find that your strengths support you or give you satisfaction or pleasure. They are things you can build on or use to move forward:

- I enjoy my job/business
- I can turn my hand to most things
- I have a happy, stable relationship and family
- I am creative
- I like to do lots of different things
- I have loads of friends

- I like change
- I have a mostly good life

What are your weaknesses?

These are things that you don't enjoy or that are bad for you – emotionally or physically. Things that you do or have in your life that probably would be better if you didn't, or if you sorted them so that they become strengths:

- I don't like working on stuff I don't like doing
- I don't like commuting
- I have no best friend to moan with since Sarah moved away
- I feel guilty about leaving the children with the minder while I work
- I want recognition
- It's hard to find time for just me and my partner without the kids
- I don't like criticism – especially from my new boss
- I find it hard to ask for help
- I need to do lots of different things
- I get bored easily
- I moan a lot
- I can have mood swings

What are your opportunities?

These are things that you could find beneficial or useful if you had some time or determination actually to do them or work on them. They are good things that you just haven't got round to yet!

- Seeking promotion
- Training abroad
- Developing new products in business
- Finding time to introduce new things into my life personally and professionally
- Having more children
- Finding a new soul mate/best friend

What are your threats?

These are things that your really need to be aware of. Weaknesses are not too damaging because you can generally turn them into strengths with a little time and thought. But threats are something you need to be constantly aware of so that you can stop, remove or prevent them. Active work on threats needs to be done sooner rather than later so you do not suffer:

- I'm unfit
- My kids exhaust me
- I have no best friend
- I'm losing interest in my job/business as it's not new any more
- I'm worried about my health
- I need vocal support from those around me
- I get bored easily
- I hate my new boss
- I get no support from the bank
- I have cash flow problems

Once you have completed a SWOT analysis, you will have all the pieces of your jigsaw and can begin to put them together. You now have the information to:

- Build on your strengths
- Strengthen your weaknesses
- Capitalise on your opportunities
- Eliminate or guard against the threats

The mere fact that you have managed to list these areas of your life means that you have been through the process of thinking about your life as a whole – we don't often do that. Now you need to consider how some aspects of your life may affect others, and look at the areas you need to make decisions on before they become problematic or get out of control.

This may be your chance to address some problems that you have put down to 'that's just the way it is' or 'I will get around to changing that one day'. Completing your own personal analysis of the relationship you have with yourself is a great way to start to look at your relationships with others.

DETOX YOUR FAMILY LIFE, SOCIAL LIFE AND PERSONAL LIFE

Follow the steps described above and take the time to work out how you are, how you think and what is good, bad and indifferent in your life. Do you feel supported or drained? Are you growing and developing or are you stagnating? Don't worry if this feels a little selfish – it's meant to be. If you don't spend time sorting yourself out and feeling fulfilled then how can you possibly help others?

You can then use the information from your SWOT analysis to refer back to, as you complete the whole relationship programme.

TASK 1: WRITE A SHORT ANALYSIS OF YOUR FAMILY LIFE

Your family is where you come from, your roots. Your family need not necessarily be blood-related, as many people are adopted or fostered. But, for these purposes your family is the group of people who brought you up and the group of people that you bring up – your own children.

Families can be nourishing, nurturing and supportive; they can be fun and sociable, strong and understanding. They can also be nightmares!

You may have thought about starting a family and you may have ideas about how you would like your family to be around you. You may doubt your ability to support your family and you may have doubts about motherhood or fatherhood.

If you had a wonderful childhood you may think that you could never re-create this yourself. This may make you doubt your ability to take responsibility for children. This needs thinking about and you need to ask if you are being a bit tough on yourself. If you had an unhappy childhood then you may desperately want to prove that your children and family will get everything they ever want, which may not be a good thing either.

Having a family and being part of a family can be one of the most difficult things in life but we tend to accept our allotted roles because we have no choice. We were born into our family and our children are born to us. There is no choosing – we get what we get.

But you do a SWOT analysis on your family life it may put some issues into perspective. It may highlight some areas that you think you can change and it may show you just how supportive your family can be.

Strengths

- Social occasions, the uniting get-togethers
- Siblings to talk about things with
- Family history, a sense of continuity
- Sense of belonging to a bigger group
- Growing family and satisfaction from watching this
- Unconditional love from parents
- Ready-made friends
- Having children continues this down the family

Weaknesses

- Having to prove yourself against brothers and sisters
- Having to stay friends even when cross with them
- Too selfish to start own family
- Not having enough time to devote to family
- Easy to think of family last, as they are always there

Opportunities

- Parties at special times of the year
- Having an information source on how to bring up a family 'on tap'
- Having children and sharing everything you have learnt with them
- Babysitting service locally supplied and trustworthy
- Satisfaction of watching sisters/brothers/parents grow and change
- Family to tell things you don't want anyone else to know
- Family that has probably experienced everything you are going through

Threats

- Fighting on issues you don't agree on
- Not being able to have children
- Children being difficult to deal with
- Not liking every member of your family
- Not always liking friends of family

The family SWOT could go on forever, depending on the extent of your family and whether you have a family or children of your own or even if you are trying for children or thinking about having children. Family SWOTs can be very funny and also be very difficult.

The one sure thing is that families are there to stay, so it is really useful to see everything about your family situation laid out in front of you. In this way, small problems that have been blown out of all proportion can be put into perspective, and larger potential problems can be headed off at the pass before they become too difficult to deal with.

If you are thinking about starting a family, you may find that there are many more strengths that you had not considered in front of you. Alternatively, there may be many more weaknesses and threats than you had thought about, while dreaming of giving birth to several perfect, quiet children that sleep and gurgle at the right time.

Getting a healthy balance of strengths, weaknesses, opportunities and threats within your own family is really important because it makes you aware of everything you need to know in order to live with your family forever and in peace!

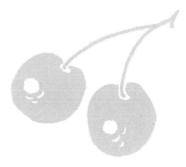

TASK 2: WRITE AN ANALYSIS OF YOUR SOCIAL LIFE

If you are ever in a personal relationship and you are treated badly or your partner takes you for granted then people usually advise you to 'finish it before someone gets hurt'. You are generally considered foolish if you don't take immediate action.

Yet, if the same is happening with a friendship, we don't seem to follow the same advice. In order to detox your life of unwanted and unproductive relationships, you should take exactly the same approach with so-called friends. Carrying out a SWOT of your friends will help you decide if the friend who has always caused you problems or heartache should now become simply an acquaintance.

Good friends can help you through the most wonderful and the most terrible of times. You can build a relationship with a friend that will provide all the support you'll ever need in your life: someone to be happy with, someone to cry with, someone to shop with, someone to do absolutely nothing with, someone to complain to, and someone to 'be the first to know'.

> **If you have good friends, and are a good friend yourself, there is little need for much else.**

Then there are friends that don't do any of the above, friends who just seem to drain you and always take without replenishing. We can all take from our friends but if this isn't eventually balanced by letting them take from you then the relationship becomes uneven and one-sided – only beneficial to one of the parties. It can even end up being detrimental to your health and happiness.

This type of friend has to go, or at least you have to be aware of what they can do to you. And you need to protect yourself from the down-side so that you can concentrate on the beneficial side to the relationship.

Doing a SWOT analysis on your friends can be difficult; simply putting names into the categories of Strengths, Weaknesses, Opportunities and Threats doesn't work. To see how your friends really measure up, you need to do a SWOT on what you need from friends and acquaintances, what you give and take from people you know, and then see who can deliver against your criteria, and who doesn't fit into any of the categories.

Doing this SWOT will demonstrate what type of friend you are and what type of friends you have. Then you can decide whether to keep things the same or to change the bits you are not quite so keen on.

Strengths

- Supportive when something goes wrong
- Can give unconditional friendship
- Enjoy lots of company
- Quite positive
- Willing to help out
- Quite broad-minded
- Not easily shocked

Weaknesses

- Don't take criticism easily
- Don't like cancellations
- Talk about myself a lot
- Always try to find experiences I have had to compare
- Want people to like me
- Say yes to helping everyone all the time
- Spend time with × but don't really like her

Opportunities

- Can make friends easily
- Can learn to take criticism
- Can listen more

Threats

- Tend to dislike at first and then get to like
- Don't like meeting new people much
- Don't always trust my instincts – try to give benefit of the doubt

Once you have completed your personal friendship SWOT, you can begin to see how your friends fill your needs and how you fill theirs. It may become clear that there are some people in your life that just cannot seem to fit in at any point and that you cannot put their name against any of your SWOT to balance you out. They drain you mentally, they only ever call when they want to talk and then they drone on about themselves.

It is now time to decide how to move forward. You may decide that a particular friend or acquaintance does so much harm and puts you down so much that you're never going to call them again. Then, if the relationship filters out, that is a positive thing. You have cleared out a negative person from your life.

Equally, you may decide that you should see some of your friends much more often because you work really well together and you get a real buzz from seeing them. They may not be the best 'match' as a friend but you may see that they counter all your bad points so you can improve by spending more time enjoying each other's company.

There may be other friends who are perfect 'matches' so be aware of this and see how you can nurture each other. If you hadn't noticed what good listeners they were, talk to them more and see where that goes.

Your SWOT may also show that you have a friend who positively drives you bananas. Now you can see why – they are probably directly opposite to you in what they bring to a relationship. This is a great finding which can help you understand that special relationship and just get on with it. You will never change each other but your unusual friendship will make much more sense.

Don't keep a friendship that upsets you or damages you – that is not a real friendship. There are plenty of people you need to deal with on a day-to-day basis that you don't like or wouldn't choose to have as a friend. So take the opportunity to change the situation and spend less and less time with someone who doesn't make your life better and more positive.

TASK 3: WRITE AN ANALYSIS OF YOUR PERSONAL RELATIONSHIP

This is the relationship with the person closest to you – whether partner or friend. Your personal relationship SWOT will actually look remarkably similar to your friendship SWOT. The qualities required in a friendship are the same as those in a personal relationship because friendship is one of the most important elements of a partnership.

If your personal relationship is going well then you probably won't feel that you need to complete this SWOT, but do it anyway because there may be room for improvement or new things that come to light. You may find that you can contribute more to the relationship. You may find out that you've been taking your partner for granted. Try putting in some extra effort and see how fabulous it can be! Don't always see SWOT analysis from your own point of view. See it from the other person's point of view as well and you may surprise yourself.

Relationships are brilliant when they are going well – fulfilling, invigorating, refreshing, pleasing, wonderful, freeing, educational and much, much more. When they aren't going well they're just plain bad. They drain you, frustrate you, upset you, anger you – and they are clearly bad for your health.

We stay in bad relationships longer than we need to. We wait for something to change and start going better without making much effort. Or we make loads of effort and there is still no change.

But if you take the time to really look at your relationship then you should be in a position to decide whether you need to finish it or move it on to the next stage.

First you need to know what you want out of a relationship. If you don't know that then how can you possibly know if it is going well or not?

Doing a SWOT on your personal life isn't about making a wish list of qualities you think your ideal partner should possess. It means becoming aware of how a very important part of your life should be going. It isn't an excuse to run away when things aren't quite going according to plan. But it does give you the chance to see what is happening and then to decide if you are happy with the situation or not, and what your next move should be.

Strengths

- I love my partner
- I get love back
- We are a team
- We go to lots of places together
- I can see that we have a future
- We like doing things together
- We are stronger together than apart

Weaknesses

- I don't have as much time for my friends
- We don't enjoy the same hobbies
- We eat different foods
- We sometimes get complacent
- I nag too much
- I do lots of housework

Opportunities

- Do lots more together
- Spend the rest of our lives together
- Develop some interest we can both share
- Learn from my partner
- Use my partner for support and help
- Use my partner to give me confidence to tackle anything

Threats

- Taking each other for granted
- Not making the effort when we should
- Getting into a rut
- Not surprising each other
- Not calling each other for a chat
- Not sharing everyday situations or problems
- Not giving each other space
- Not making sure we share quality time

After completing your personal relationship SWOT you should find things that *both* of you can do. If you only find that there are things that your partner should be doing for you then you should revisit the Threats section and put in there that you always assume you are right. This is a threat because if you believe it then you are probably fooling yourself. And if you are not fooling yourself then maybe there are some areas you have forgotten to include.

There may be things that will just improve the balance in every area of your relationship and there may well be things on which you need to make a really specific effort in order to save the relationship. You may decide that you want to open this section up to your partner. Get them to complete their own SWOT, and then make the time and go through the results together. You never know – there could be things you do without thinking that drive your partner wild with happiness or mad with frustration!

There may be things that have been festering away . . . Now is the time to meet them head on. And there may be other things that you can look at and deal with before they ever get the chance to become an issue.

Get personal and detox all your relationships right now! If you know you want to work together, play together and live together then surely it is worth investing some time to change things for the better.

User's Manual

This resource section contains extra information that may be useful when following the different detox programmes described in the book.

The information is listed in the same order as the programmes.

THE 30-DAY ULTIMATE DETOX

LIST OF PERMITTED FOODS FOR THE FOOD PROGRAMME

Fruit

Choose any dried or fresh fruits from the following:

Apples	Greengages	Paw-paw
Apricots	Guavas	Peaches
Bilberries	Kiwi fruit	Pears
Blackberries	Lemons	Pineapples
Cherries	Limes	Plums
Cranberries	Loganberries	Pomegranates
Currants	Lychees	Prunes
Damsons	Mangoes	Quinces
Dates	Melons	Raisins
Figs	Mulberries	Raspberries
Gooseberries	Nectarines	Rhubarb
Grapefruit	Olives (green or black)	Strawberries
Grapes	Passion fruit	Sultanas

Vegetables

Artichokes (globe or Jerusalem)	Cauliflower	Parsnips
	Celeriac	Peas (all types)
Asparagus	Celery	Peppers
Aubergines	Chicory	Plantains
Bean sprouts	Chinese leaf	Potatoes
Beans (French, runner, broad, butter, haricot, mung, red kidney)	Courgettes	Pumpkin
	Cucumber	Radishes
	Fennel	Spring greens
	Kohlrabi	Swedes
Beetroot	Leeks	Sweetcorn
Broccoli	Lettuce (all types)	Sweet potatoes
Brussel sprouts	Marrow	Squash
Cabbage (red, Savoy, spring, white, winter)	Okra	Turnips
	Onions	Watercress
Carrots	Parsley	Yams

Nuts

Almonds	Chestnuts	Pecan
Brazil	Hazel	Pine
Cashew	Macadamia	Walnuts

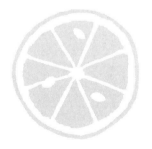

Pulses, seeds, herbs and spices

Alfalfa	Dill	Pumpkin seeds
Basil	Fennel	Rosemary
Cardamom pods	Ginger (fresh and	Sage
Cayenne pepper	ground)	Sesame seeds
Chickpeas	Marjoram	Sunflower seeds
Chilli (ground)	Parsley	Tarragon
Chillies (fresh)	Pepper (fresh,	Thyme
Coriander	ground)	

Non-dairy products

Goat's cheese	Sheep's milk	Soya milk
Sheep's cheeses	Goat's yoghurt	Rice milk
Goat's milk	Sheep's yoghurt	

Fish

Cod	Lobster	Sardines
Crab	Mackerel	Scampi
Haddock	Pilchards	Shrimps
Halibut	Plaice	Skate
Herring	Prawns	Trout
Lemon Sole	Salmon	Tuna

Drinks

Water (hot, cold, fizzy, spring, tap)

Herbal teas (any)

Lemon juice in water

Honey in water

Juices (freshly squeezed, pure and unsweetened, apple or grape or any juiced vegetable)

Note

If you are buying ready-squeezed juices, go for pure juice rather than the juice made up from a concentrate – it will say on the carton or bottle. If you find the juice too strong, dilute to taste with water. This makes the juice go further *and* increases your water intake.

Miscellaneous

Olive oil	Apple cider vinegar	Tofu
Olives	Balsamic vinegar	Quorn
Sesame oil	Miso	Brown rice
Grapeseed oil	Mustard (grain not	Rice cakes (unsalted)
Walnut oil	powder)	Seaweed
	Tahini	

Note

Tahini can be bought from most healthfood stores. You can use 'light' tahini (for which the sesame seeds are hulled before being ground) or 'dark' tahini (which simply means that the hulls have been left on). Make sure that your tahini is unsalted. Most are but it's worth checking the ingredients.

List of foods you definitely cannot have and why

Avocados	Too much starch and fat
Bananas	Too much starch and fat
Bread	Gluten in wheatflour can be difficult to digest
Caffeine	Chemical stimulant
Chocolate	Too much sugar and fat
Cow's milk, cheese, etc	Lactose (milk sugar) can be difficult to digest
Lentils	Too much gas
Mushrooms	Too much fungus
Oranges	Too acidic
Peanuts	Too much fat and starch
Salt	Too much salt results in potassium deficiency and water retention
Spinach	Too acidic
Sugar	Disturbs blood glucose levels, causing disturbed appetite and energy levels
Tomatoes	Too acidic

As you can see, the 'forbidden' list is very short and the choice of available foods on the Ultimate Detox programme is extensive, so there is absolutely no excuse to stray. Following these lists will still enable you to prepare very interesting and varied meals. In fact you may enjoy eating this way so much that you decide to stick to it permanently!

The mind programme

Affirmations

Affirmations are a brilliant way of feeling good about yourself immediately, and they have long-term benefits as well. Feeling down in the dumps can be transformed into feeling positive and pro-active in just a matter of moments. And when you have got into the habit of saying your own affirmations, feeling down in the dumps becomes a thing of the past.

During the Ultimate Detox you can affirm your ability to complete the programme and you can visualise just how 'clean' you will be when you have finished.

Whether you have completed the detox, whether you are thinking about beginning it, or just about any other time in your life, you can use affirmations to help you.

You often hear people say – 'and if someone tells you this often enough, you really start to believe them'. Well that's all that affirmations are: telling yourself something, anything, often enough that you really believe it. And if you believe something then it becomes real.

Affirmations don't have to be grand or extraordinary, they just have to help you. To start making affirmations you need to think about what you want to happen or what you want to do. It can be on any level: personal, job, home, relationship, money – anything. It is probably better to start with something small. Giving up your job and living on a tropical island might be a little too adventurous for starters! And, anyway, if you change something small it almost always leads to something bigger.

Affirmations must be positive and should be kept short. The sorts of things you might want to affirm during your Ultimate Detox would be:

- I have a healthy body
- I am happy with my body

- I am cleaning my body
- This is my month, I will enjoy looking after myself
- I deserve to indulge myself this month
- I am feeling great
- I am feeling energetic
- I have succeeded with my own personal detox.

You get the idea . . . Now all you have to do is repeat these to yourself or out loud. You should say them whenever they come into your mind. You can say all of them or just one of them. As you are saying your affirmations you should give them positive energy: feel good about saying them and smile whilst you are saying them. You should believe that they are real, they exist and that they have come true or are coming true for you. If there is a time when you say your affirmations and you feel same doubt or negativity, say them again immediately – this time with all the positive belief you can muster.

If you find it difficult to remember your affirmations just jot them down on the bottom of your 'to do' list, your shopping list or your diary. Then, each time you see them, say them to yourself two or three times.

Affirmations are completely personal. No one needs to hear them or even know that you make them. The only rule is that they have to be exactly what you want. Here are some examples:

- I deserve more money
- I am going to get a better job
- I am great
- I am fun to be with
- I am going to ask him/her out
- I will tell him/her that I don't agree
- I will have more time for myself
- I won't let them get to me
- I am successful in everything I do.

The body programme

Dry skin brushing

Now that you have read about all the excellent reasons to dry skin brush, the next step is to learn how to do it effectively:

- Find a natural bristle brush or loofah or a dry flannel or mitt. The brush, loofah or mitt should be firm but not hard. You will be brushing the skin all over your body quite vigorously – and the skin on your stomach is softer than the skin on your shins or forearms. Do not wet or moisturise the skin, as this may cause dragging.

- Having undressed to your underwear, or preferably with no clothes on, stand or sit in a position that gives you access to all parts of your body. The edge of the bed with feet on pillows is quite good, or you could sit on the edge of the bath with one foot up on the toilet seat.

- Start at your feet and systematically work up towards the top of your body. All strokes should be towards your heart (venous return). The heart does a wonderful job of pumping the blood down throughout the body, but both blood and lymph need extra help to work against gravity to return through the system. If you brush away from the heart it may cause faintness or disrupt the normal flow. Each stroke should be long and firm. Place the brush/mitt on your ankle and firmly brush up to the knee. Repeat several times until you have covered the entire calf and shin several times. When you have completed the lower leg, move up to the knee. The next strokes should run from the knee to the top of the thigh and over the buttocks.

- Then brush both arms, from the wrist to the shoulder. The neck and shoulder area should be treated more gently as the flesh here is very delicate. Work from the top of the arm, up and over the shoulder and gently up the neck to the base of the skull.

- When brushing the stomach, use gentle circular strokes in a clockwise direction. This will follow the flow in your intestines and will not disrupt bowel functions.

Note

You must only brush the face with a soft facial brush or flannel as facial skin is very delicate and can be damaged if the brush is too hard.

EXERCISE SEQUENCE

- Walk up and down ten steps or stairs for 5 minutes at a normal pace.

- Stand with your feet shoulder-width apart. Alternately lift your left leg and left arm up and out to the side, then your right leg and right arm up and out to the side. Repeat 10 times each side. NB: Keep your arms and knees slightly bent.

- Standing in the same position, clasp your hands in front of your nose with your arms slightly bent. Keeping your shoulders relaxed, twist slowly, from side to side. The stretch will increase gradually, and you should end it when you can see directly behind yourself. Feel the stretch in your stomach and waist muscles. Repeat 10 times each side.

- Walk on the spot for 5 minutes, making sure that you bring each knee up to hip level. Swing your arms up and down in a marching motion – bring your hands up to shoulder height.

- Walk on the spot for 5 minutes bringing your knees up to hip level. Now clasp your hands in front of you with your forearms close together. As you step, lift your arms and lower them. (Do not let your arms drop below shoulder height.)

- Jog on the spot for 5 minutes without lifting your toes from the floor. You are just lifting your heels up and down and wiggling your hips as much as possible.

- Facing forward, twist your head slowly from side to side, and look over your right and left shoulder alternately. Hold the stretch for a moment, release and then look over the other shoulder.

- Standing with your feet shoulder-width apart, hold the back of an upright chair and lower your body down until your knees are bent at a 90-degree angle. Hold the position for a count of five and lift up slowly. Repeat 15 times. Remember to clench your buttocks and thighs as you lift and lower your body.

- Kneel on the floor with your hands shoulder-width apart, flat on the floor. 'Walk' your hands forward so that you are leaning your body weight onto your hands and using your knees as a balance.

Keeping your back straight, bend and lower your arms until your nose touches the floor and then lift – repeat 10 times, slowly.

RELAXATION SEQUENCE

Find a quiet room, make sure you are warm and choose some melodic, peaceful music.

- Lie down on the floor or sit comfortably in a chair.

- Close your eyes and start to breathe deeply as described in the breathing exercise below.

- After breathing correctly for a couple of minutes you should find that your breathing has slowed down and this will feel very natural.

- When you inhale, imagine that the air you are breathing is warm and golden and is bathing your body in warm, golden, restful, positive light.

- Now start to consider how your body is feeling. As you inhale, start thinking about your feet and ankles. Are they tense? If so, relax them.

- As you exhale, picture the air you breathe out as old stagnant air, and the air you breathe in as new, fresh air.

- Think of your calves and knees. Picture the warm air travelling through any tense muscles, bathing them in light. Exhale the stale air.

- Picture your knee joints and your upper leg area. Breathe deeply and relax.

- Feel the air being breathed into the groin area, relaxing the tension and soothing the pelvis. Breathe out the bad air.

- See the golden light swirling around your stomach and abdomen, cleansing and uplifting your centre of emotion and spirit.

- Watch the light thread its way between each and every rib, filling your lungs and chest cavity with warm expanding air.

- Watch each and every finger fill with golden light and spread through your hands and lower arms.

- Breathe the energy into your shoulders and the base of your neck. Feel your neck relax and melt into the floor and up into the base of your skull.

- The light may now travel into the root of each and every hair follicle, making your scalp feel invigorated and tingling.

- Each time you exhale you are breathing out waste. Each time you breathe in you are breathing in new life.

- When you have renewed the life inside your body you should look to see where the source of your new breath and new light is coming from.

- With your eyes still closed, look above you and see the beam of light coming down towards your body. See it feeding into your abdomen. You are connected to this light and you can take as much as you wish.

- Breathe deeply and inhale all you need.

- When you are ready you can start to think about bringing your consciousness back into your own body and into the room you are in.

- Open your eyes slowly. If you are lying on the floor or bed, roll over onto your side and wait a few moments before you eventually push yourself up to a sitting and then to a standing position.

You should now feel totally relaxed and invigorated. Well done!

BREATHING

This is a good breathing exercise to do when you feel stressed or if you cannot sleep or if you simply want to recharge your batteries:

BREATHING EXERCISE

- Sit comfortably or lie down – supporting your lower back if necessary.

- Place your hands on your stomach area with the fingertips just touching.

- Start to breathe in through your nose very slowly to a count of four. (As you inhale, you should feel your stomach expand and your fingertips separate.)

- Hold the breath for four and exhale slowly through your mouth to a count of eight.

- Repeat several times as required.

It will feel strange at first, as you are not used to using your muscles to expand your stomach in this way. But after just a few minutes it will start to feel more natural.

Continue this exercise for at least ten inward breaths and you should feel much more relaxed and 'centred'. Eventually you will not need to use your fingers to check that your stomach (rather than your chest) is expanding. And soon you will be able to carry out this exercise whilst you are going about your normal day-to-day business – not the lying down but the controlled breathing! If you ever have difficulty dropping off to sleep, this is a far more effective solution than the traditional 'counting sheep'. The chances are that you won't even make it to ten – you will probably be asleep by six.

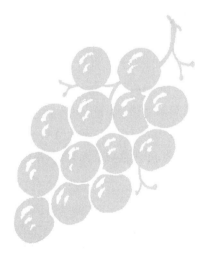

> ### Home-made exfoliating scrub mix
> (Makes enough for one bath/scrub)
>
> 1 tablespoon salt flakes (you can use normal salt if your skin
>   is delicate or you want a less rigorous product)
> 2 tablespoons olive, vegetable or seed oil (e.g. sunflower,
>   sesame, etc)
> 1 tablespoon thick honey
> A few drops of fennel or peppermint essential oil
>
> Place all the ingredients in a plastic bowl and mix together until
> you have a runny paste.
>
> Dip the ends of your fingers into the pot and scoop out
> about a teaspoon of the mixture each time. Rub this all over
> your body and apply more when required. (The salt is the
> exfoliant, the oil and honey will help to moisturise the flesh, and
> the essential oils will stimulate digestion and detox.)

Alternatively, you can turn your favourite body oil into an exfoliant by simply adding the salt to a small amount of your chosen product and then use as described below.

You can exfoliate in the bath or shower, but unless you have a palatial shower you may find that the cream has been washed off before you get the chance to benefit from its exfoliating properties! Ideally you should exfoliate during a nice relaxing bath. Here's how:

DIY EXFOLIATION

- Run a bath and put a few drops of your favourite bath oil or
  foam into the water. Get in and relax!

- Allow at least 10 minutes before you start to exfoliate. This will give you time to relax and your skin time to soften with the water/oils etc. You now have two options.

- *Either* get out of the bath, making sure the bathroom is still nice and warm, and gently rub your exfoliating cream or home-made exfoliant in firm, large and small circles all over your body. Pay special attention to any areas of hard skin (heels, knees, elbows, etc) and rub as hard as you find comfortable. The whole process should take about 3–4 minutes. When you have completed the 'rub', get back into the bath and carry on the circular rubbing until all the cream has been washed off into the bath water. Get out of the bath and then rub yourself dry with a towel. (Use a towel that has not been rinsed in fabric conditioner as this will increase its absorbency and will carry on the exfoliating process as you are drying yourself.) Once dry, apply a good moisturiser or body oil all over your body and stay warm. Going to bed with a good book, for an early night, is definitely the best option!

- *Or* stay in the bath, lift each limb above the surface of the water, and exfoliate as described above, in firm, large and small circles. As you finish each limb, lower it back into the water and continue to work the flesh until all the cream has been washed away. The only area that may get neglected using this method is the buttocks but you can do this area by kneeling up in the bath. Towel dry as above, then moisturise and keep warm.

EPSOM SALTS BATHING

Run a deep bath that is warm enough to sit in for 10 or 15 minutes without going cold or being too hot to sit in. Pour about 1 kg (2 lb) Epsom salts (available from most chemists or healthfood stores) into your bath and stir until it has all dissolved. It *is* a lot but you need this much to get the best effect. Get into the bath and have ready some sort of glove or massage mitt.

Sit in the bath for at least 5 minutes before you start to massage your body. Start massaging with slow gentle strokes; as you get more used to this, make the strokes more rigorous. It is likely that you will feel very warm quite quickly as the magnesium has a warming effect. If this happens, slow down your massage and just let the Epsom salts work on you as you relax.

When you get out of the bath you should pat yourself dry and then wrap up warm for the next hour or so. Ideally you should take the bath in the evening just before you are about to go to bed. This will keep you warm for many hours. Alternatively, you can take the bath during the day, wrap up in a quilt or blanket and sit and watch an old movie!

Don't be surprised if you feel quite tired after an Epsom bath as it will be having quite an effect on your internal systems — all for the good.

Important Note
Do *not* take an Epsom salt bath if you suffer from any skin condition or if you have any cuts or grazes.

AROMATHERAPY

When taking on the task of detoxing, you should use all the support and help you can get.

Aromatherapy and essential oils are one of the ways that you can have this support with you at all times and the only evidence to anyone that you are using them is that you will smell nice!

> **Important Note**
>
> Essential oils should never be used if you believe you are pregnant
> or if you are trying to become pregnant unless otherwise
> prescribed by a trained aromatherapist. Essential oils should never
> be taken internally.

The use of aromatherapy oils is recorded as early as 3000 BC. The Egyptians used oils for medical and cosmetic purposes as well as for embalming. The Greeks and Romans used them in medical practice, and medieval documents include many references to scented oils.

During the eighteenth and nineteenth centuries, substances such as morphine, caffeine and quinine were recorded as ingredients obtained from medicinal plants. And in the present day we still use plant extracts (e.g. lavender and peppermint) in common drugs.

It should also be pointed out that some of the most dangerous drugs available today are still those derived from the plant family: e.g. heroin, cannabis, arsenic and digitalis.

Aromatherapy oils are therefore not to be taken lightly. They can be dangerous if used incorrectly or in the wrong amounts. They are not just nice-smelling oils, as some people believe, but strong, effective drugs that can have both subtle and huge effects on the body, mind and emotions. They should always be used with caution and treatment should be under the supervision of a qualified aromatherapist or by following instructions in a book or leaflet. You should never just choose an oil because it smells nice. It may have side-effects or contra-indications that could be harmful or dangerous.

There are hundreds of essential oils available. Many should be left to the professional practitioner but there are a few that you may wish to use at home for your own detox programme. Be sure to follow the instructions on how to use oils at home when bathing, inhaling, or carrying out self-massage. Please remember that these oils are incredibly strong and should always be used diluted unless under qualified advice and direction.

Aromatherapy/essential oils and bathing

Essential oils should never be used for bathing or massage without being first diluted in base or carrier oils, or dispersed in a substance that will break the oil down.

Dispersants can be found in the house and the two most readily available are milk or high-volume alcohol (vodka is best as it has no fragrance and no sugar residue). These products will break down the essential oil into much smaller droplets which will mean the oil is more evenly spread in the water and is less likely to cause irritation to your skin.

Diluting your essential oil with a base or carrier oil will make your bath more oily. This is great when you can massage the residue of oil into your skin after the bath. But if you are bathing first thing in the morning, or if you need to dress immediately after the bath, then a dispersant is more practical as it will immediately absorb into your skin after the bath without leaving any greasy residue.

When bathing in oils you should not attempt to use any soap or gel for washing, as this will destroy the effects of the natural oil. Choose a time when you do not need to wash (i.e. just before bed or after you have taken a quick shower). Run a bath that is hot enough to stay warm for 15–20 minutes but not so hot that it is uncomfortable to sit in.

Decide whether to dilute or disperse your essential oil in order to make up your blend. You only need a tablespoon of dispersant or carrier oil. Then add 2–4 drops of essential oil to this.

Essential oil bath

- When the bath is full, let the water go calm. Then sprinkle a tablespoon of your blended oil over the water.

- Close all the windows so that none of the steam escapes. You might also want to light some candles to create a really relaxing sensuous experience. Slowly get into the bath, and, once in, concentrate on breathing slowly and deeply, inhaling all the vapour of the oil. Allow your skin to soak and absorb all the oils. You should be able to totally relax and unwind. Try to healthy mind detox!

- Once you have finished your bath, get out slowly. If you have used a carrier oil try to collect all the oil from the surface of the water onto your skin. Pat yourself dry, allowing as much of the oil as possible to stay on your flesh, acting as a natural moisturiser and allowing any residual oil to continue to be absorbed. Even if you have used a dispersant there will still be a small amount of oil to massage into your skin. If you need to dress after your bath you should be able to let the oil absorb as you would a body cream or moisturiser.

- Ideally you can now relax or go straight to bed.

Aromatherapy/essential oils and inhalations

Using essential oils for inhalations is an excellent and very quick way to benefit from them.

When you breathe in the vapour from the oils it enters the olfactory system instantly so attention should be paid to the amount of oil used. As with many natural therapies, correct dosage will solve a problem but using too much will often worsen the same problem.

Rather like any 'grandmother's remedy' you need to boil some water and pour it into a large bowl. Add 2–3 drops of your chosen oil – no dispersants or carriers are required as the oil does not come into direct contact with your skin – and lower your head, covered with a towel or sheet, over the bowl. As you inhale slowly through your nose and out through your mouth you can lower your face closer to the water as you become used to the vapour. Inhaling is an excellent method for colds and coughs, as the effects are immediate and relief is very welcome. Inhale for about 5 minutes or until you have had enough. Then uncover your head and breathe the cool air.

You can also inhale oils by placing 2–3 drops on an old handkerchief (the oils may stain). Holding the cloth near your nose or mouth, you can inhale in the same way. Do not hold the cloth directly on your skin as the oils may irritate.

Aromatherapy/essential oils and compresses

There are some times when nothing more than a hot-water bottle is required to relieve discomfort or pain or simply to give warmth and comfort. Using a compress is the aromatherapy answer to this.

You need to fill a large bowl with hand-hot water, add 2–3 drops of your chosen essential oil to the water and soak a large piece of cotton cloth for a couple of minutes. Then you need to wring out the cloth and fold it into a compress large enough to cover the area of discomfort, i.e. a 15 cm (6 inch) square. Add 2 further drops of your oil directly onto the compress (it will spread and dilute into the soaked cotton), then hold the compress onto the area of pain. You can use the compress until it cools down, and if you wish you can repeat the process.

An essential oil compress is ideal for period pains, fever and headaches as the oil can be applied directly, in a soothing relaxing way, though you can, of course, use a compress for any condition or any reason. For instance, if you get the chance just to sit down and relax then a nice Lavender and Ylang Ylang compress (both oils for relaxation and rejuvenation) would make the 5 minutes even more relaxing!

Aromatherapy/essential oils and burners

Using oil burners is an excellent way of getting essential oils into the atmosphere so that you can benefit from their therapeutic qualities whilst you go about your everyday business. NB: Oils should not be used when there are children under five in the room or house.

The choice of burner is quite important as there are many available on the market that look wonderful but are not very practical. When choosing your burner you need to get one with a bowl that is big enough to contain 120 ml (4 oz) water. If the bowl holds much more than this then it will take too long to heat the water; and if the bowl is much smaller then it will have burnt dry, giving a rancid smell, before the candle has gone out. You need to fill the burner with water, light the candle below and then drop 4–5 drops of your chosen oil onto the surface of the water. You are unlikely to use too much oil in a burner, as the vapour is distributed throughout the entire building. But if you start to develop a mild headache simply add more water or blow out the candle.

The alternative is to use dry burners – the terracotta rings that go on light bulbs, or the electrically heated porcelain plates. These work by putting a few drops of your chosen oil onto the heated surface. The heat releases the vapour, and they can be controlled by turning off the power or removing the terracotta burner.

Aromatherapy/essential oils and ready-made blends

We have 'fast' everything now and ready-made blends are the complementary therapy answer to using essential oils quickly, relatively inexpensively and safely.

If people decide to use essential oils at home after reading a short book about them, they run the risk of causing quite a lot of damage. It is human nature to add your own personal interpretation to anything you read, but when using essential oils, any interpretation or creativity can be dangerous. When baking a cake you might decide to add more orange zest than the recipe suggests to boost the flavour and colour – this is likely to do both things successfully and therefore make your cake even more delicious. But if you were to apply the same method in creating an essential oil blend – perhaps adding more Basil because you like the smell – then your blend could take on a completely different quality and might well worsen the problem rather than solving it. Essential oils tend to work on the same principle as many natural remedies: 'a little will cure and a lot will cause'.

Ready-made blends are therefore an excellent way to introduce yourself to aromatherapy without any risk of getting it wrong. There are, however, a few guidelines you should follow in order to get the best out of your oils.

Coloured oils

About 99 per cent of essential oils are a clear light yellow colour. Some go as far as deep orange (e.g. Neroli and Mandarin) and some are very light, almost non-coloured (e.g. Lavender). Very few, and certainly very uncommon oils, are what we would call coloured – Blue Camomile is an incredibly dark blue, almost ink-like colour. So it is fair to say that most of the oils you would come across for day-to-day use are light yellow. Carrier or base oils are the same. They are all varying degrees of yellow to mid-brown. Grapeseed is slightly greener and nut oils are very dark brown but all are fairly neutral.

So if you look at the products available in shops, their colour will tell you how natural they are, and how much of the essential oil they actually contain. For instance, if you pick a blend for massage containing Lavender and other relaxing oils then the blend should be a neutral colour, not bright blue or dark green. If you want a bath oil to invigorate you then a bright pink or orange one is only likely to perk you up if you look at it rather than bathe in it! This is not to say that there is no place for these products. It is great that people are being made more aware of the properties of aromatherapy oils and they make wonderful gifts. If they encourage you to take a bath or have a massage then that has many benefits in itself. However, if you wish to use essential oils for their specific, therapeutic qualities then you really need to use the pure essential oil in a carrier or base oil.

Oils for detox

There are many, many essential oils available on the market today. The following list includes oils that are particularly helpful when detoxing.

- **Juniper** is an astringent, antiseptic, detoxifying oil. It is often used as a tonic oil, as it can help to speed up a sluggish circulation and increase elimination. Juniper is a diuretic and will therefore increase the expulsion of toxins and waste through urine. It speeds up the metabolic rate which increases the detox rate. As a 'cleansing' oil, it works on both a physical and emotional level, detoxing the mind and the body.

- **Fennel** is great for the digestion and strengthens peristalsis (the contraction of the intestinal muscles). Fennel is also a diuretic which helps prevents water retention. Fennel is an antiseptic that works in the urinary tract and kidneys, protecting them from germs and maintaining a favourable environment during detox. Fennel is a general tonic, helping to increase circulation and remove waste and toxins.

- **Rosemary** is one of the best 'all-round' essential oils. It is a great balancer of moods and physical manifestations. It has a wonderfully stimulating effect on the central nervous system and the rest of the body and is one of the best oils to use as a natural 'pick-me-up'. Rosemary is a tonic for the heart, skin, kidneys, spleen and blood; it stimulates circulation and boosts low blood pressure. NB: Rosemary should not be used in cases of epilepsy.

- **Lemongrass** is a cleansing and refreshing oil. As a spicy oil, it stimulates the digestion and eases nervous stomach conditions. It promotes the removal of toxins from the body and is antiseptic and bactericidal.

- **Peppermint** is used as a remedy for digestive problems and helps the stomach, liver and intestines. Peppermint will ease any strain placed on the intestines and stomach during detox and will decrease swelling and bloating. Peppermint can also be used to stimulate the mind! Peppermint is cooling and relaxing and is often used in stomach pills and cooling leg or foot balms.

- **Pine** is best used for inhalations or in burners, as it is a very strong oil. Pine is refreshing and uplifting. It has a stimulating effect on the circulation and helps to remove any phlegm or mucous conditions caused by detoxing.

- **Basil** stimulates the brain and uplifts the mind! Basil has been used for stomach complaints and can help with the digestive system during detox. Basil boosts confidence and increases low energy. It enhances the circulation but is very potent so it should be used sparingly.

The following oils are also good for detox but more specifically for the Healthy Mind Detox:

- **Rose** is one of the most expensive but also one of the most amazing and magical oils. Rose has anti-inflammatory properties and is great for any 'feminine' conditions such as PMS, anorexia, self-loathing and stomach cramps. This is a real treat and incredibly beneficial.

- **Geranium** balances. If you are hyper it calms you down and if you are down it perks you up. Ideal for hormone imbalance, depression and general mood swings.

- **Eucalyptus** 'will kill all known germs, dead'. So when you are feeling at a low ebb, kick in with this oil and feel the benefits. It will also stimulate and invigorate and banish the nasty itching caused by insect bites and stings.

- **Camomile** will relax the mind and body. It has a calming effect physically and mentally and will help you to sleep through the night in order to continue detoxing your life with renewed vigour the next day.

THE WEEKEND DETOX

JUICING AND SMOOTHIES

Juicing is using just the juice of a combination of fruits and/or vegetables.

Smoothies can be a combination of fruits with yoghurt, ice cream, cream or any other thickening agent like fruit pulp or soya milk.

There are just a few rules with both juicing and smoothies to ensure that you get a fabulous fruity/veggie cocktail of your choosing. As long as you observe these, you can let your imagination run wild:

- Always wash every fruit/vegetable you blend or juice.

- Make sure your fruit/vegetable is both fresh and ripe.

- Blend just one or two fruits and vegetables at a time. Mixing a crazy concoction may result in green gunge that puts you off the whole idea!

- Wash your juicer/blender every time it is used.

Suggested beginners' juices:

Fruits	Vegetables
Apples	Beetroot
Bananas	Carrots
Blackcurrants	Celery
Grapefruit	Cucumber
Grapes	Ginger root – a little for taste
Lemons	Spinach
Melon	Watercress
Oranges	
Peaches	
Pears	
Pineapple	
Plums	
Strawberries	

Here are a few more hints to get the best juices or smoothies:

- If you blend frozen fruit with ice cream or frozen plain yoghurt then you will get your own home-made frozen smoothie.

- Fruits/vegetables that are high in water content, with thin skins, can simply be placed in a normal blender, after de-seeding if required. Then blend to either a chunky or very smooth consistency. There is no need to peel them. The peel will actually add to the flavour and nutritional value of juices made from grapes, peaches, melons, strawberries, apples, blackcurrants, pears, celery, carrots and cucumber, for example.

- To get a thicker consistency, add natural, organic fruit or plain yoghurt. Add slowly to get the ideal blend and texture.

- Thicker fruits or more fibrous vegetables (e.g. oranges, grapefruit, lemons, limes, beetroot, watercress or spinach) will need to be either peeled before blending or juiced in a centrifugal juicer (one that spins the fruit pulp into a cup and discards the waste after extracting all the goodness).

- Add normal juice or water to heavy vegetable blends to make them more palatable and easier on the digestive system.

Just enjoy using your imagination and discover the delights of taking in bucketloads of goodness in one small glass.

FASTING

Fasting has been popular for many hundreds of years as a way of totally cleansing your insides. Fasting means eating nothing and drinking only water.

Fasting allows your body to get rid of waste and empty its systems of all food residues. The clearer the path, the more efficiently the body can absorb and use the nutrients you take in afterwards. Fasting also facilitates the release of hormones that stimulate the immune system.

> **Important Note**
> There are a number of different lengths of fast which can be undertaken. But if you wish to complete a fast of three days or more it must always be done under supervision. Long-term fasting – without correct supervision and instruction – can do more harm than good.

Literally 'starving' your body for more than 24 hours will lead to feelings of weakness, nausea, muscle fatigue, dehydration and dizziness. If you try to operate normally (going to work, looking after the family, etc) you are likely to experience major lapses in concentration and extreme fatigue. If you have any previous health conditions then these will be exacerbated by lack of food and nourishment.

There are other forms of fasting that are less severe and, in my view, much more effective. Restricting your diet to certain types of cleansing foods for 24–48 hours can help to maintain and/or boost the detox programme.

After you have completed your detox programme you may sometimes feel that you have eaten too many processed foods or have had to eat out a lot and don't feel as if you have been very kind to your body. At times like these you can try a mini fast. You can also think about trying a mini mini fast more regularly, perhaps once a week, on an evening when you are not going out.

If you fast after you have detoxed it will bring positive results immediately. Each time you fast you will just be flushing out a small build-up of toxins and waste. Fasting regularly after detox will therefore maintain the detox at its fullest potential.

Don't just decide to fast and starve yourself for the next few days. Preparation is essential if you wish to get the best results.

How to fast

First check that you fulfil the necessary health requirements. As with any detox programme, you must not be:

- Pregnant
- Breast-feeding
- Suffering from any illness or heart condition
- Diabetic
- Taking prescribed drugs
- Having any doubts about your personal health

Then decide when you want to fast and for how long – a mini fast (18–24 hours) or a mini, mini fast (10–14 hours).

It's important to start and finish gradually.

- For the 48 hours leading up to your fast, you should cut out caffeine, red meat, processed foods and alcohol.

- The three meals prior to your fast should be meals from the detox programme (i.e. only using ingredients from the food lists on pp. 160–4).

- Throughout the fast you should drink plenty of hot water, lemon juice and honey.

- Drink at least 1.5 litres (3 pints) of fluid, in the form of water, herbal teas, apple, grape or lemon juice, each day.

- If hunger becomes unbearable then have some black grapes at hand to nibble on.

Once you have finished your fast, you should eat only foods from the lists on pp. 160–4 for a day. Then slowly introduce normal foods in the same way as you would when finishing any detox programme.

The mini fast

The mini fast can be done once a month and will give your body the 'time out' it needs to cleanse itself internally. As the mini fast starts overnight, you are actually only aware of fasting for around 10 hours.

- The mini fast lasts from early evening to late afternoon the following day.

- Having eaten detox foods during the day, you should eat a light vegetarian meal – ideally from the detox programme – before 6.30 p.m.

- Eat *nothing* until late afternoon the following day but make sure you drink plenty of herbal teas, juices or water during the early evening and following day.

- Your first meal after your fast should be light and consist of fruit, salad and brown rice.

- At 6 p.m. have another meal of fresh fruit and vegetables.

The mini, mini fast

The mini, mini fast should be done once a week and can probably be done without really noticing you are on a fast! The mini, mini fast takes place overnight from around 6.30 p.m. to 8 a.m. the following morning.

As with the mini fast, you are actually asleep for the bulk of this fast so it feels like a short 4- or 5-hour fast. As it is so short, you may wonder why it is worth doing and how can it have any benefit. Yet even fasting for such a short time still gives your body time to process and cleanse.

Getting into the habit of eating your final meal of the day as early as possible gives your body a better chance to digest the food correctly. Whether or not you are detoxing, the benefits of proper digestion should not be underestimated.

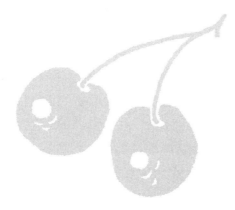

Useful Addresses

This section contains useful contact numbers and addresses for treatments and courses discussed in this book.

THE BRITISH SCHOOL OF COMPLEMENTARY THERAPY

The British School of Complementary Therapy offers a number of valuable courses and treatments:

Courses

Diplomas in Aromatherapy, Diplomas in Massage, Diplomas in Reflexology, LaStone Therapy training, Introduction to Homoeopathy, Introduction to Iridology, Indian Head Massage, Beginners' Aromatherapy Weekends and Beginners' Massage Weekends.

Treatments

Aromatherapy, Massage, Acupuncture, Reflexology, Cranio-sacral Therapy, LaStone Therapy and Thai Massage.

For further information, prospectus, treatment details and to order essential oils, please call 020 7224 2394. Or visit our website at www.bsct.co.uk or www.lastonetherapy.com

OTHER USEFUL CONTACTS

These UK organisations can help you find fully qualified, registered, practitioners in your area.

British Complementary Medicine Association
9 Soar Lane, Leicester LE3 5DE
Tel: 0116 242 5406

Institute for Complementary Medicine
PO Box 194, London SE16 1QZ
Tel: 020 7237 5165

Aromatherapy Organisations Council
3 Latymer Close, Braybrooke, Market Harborough LE16 8LN

British Acupuncture Council
Park House, 206–208 Latimer Road, London W10 6RE
Tel: 020 8964 0222

The Edward Bach Centre (Bach Flower Remedies)
Mount Vernon, Bakers Lane, Sotwell, Wallingford, OX10 OPZ
Tel: 01491 834678

Colonic International Association

16 Englands Lane, London NW3 4TG

Tel: 020 7483 1595

Kay Tom (Space Clearing Practitioner)

Leicestershire

Tel: 01509 213369

E-mail: Kay_T@compuserve.com

Available for UK consultations

Karen Kingston (Space Clearing Practitioner)

Suite 401, Langham House, 29 Margaret Street, London W1N 7LB

Tel: 07000 772232

E-mail: ukoffice@spaceclearing.com

Association of Reflexologists

27 Old Gloucester Street, London WC1 3XX

Tel: 0990 673320

Roger Coghill (Reading material on Electromagnetic Stress)

Coghill Research Laboratories, Lower Race, Pontypool, Gwent NP4 5UH

Tel: 01495 752122

Transcendental Meditation

Freepost, London SW1P 4YY

Tel: 08705 143733

Yoga for Health Foundation

Ickwell Bury, Ickwell Green, Biggleswade, Bedfordshire SG18 9EF

Tel: 01767 627271

The School of Feng Shui (Feng Shui Courses and Information)
2 Cherry Orchard, Shipston on Stour, Warwickshire CV36 4QR
Tel: 01608 664998
www.fengshui-school.co.uk
E-mail: info@fengshui-school.co.uk

The Soil Association (Information on Organic Food Suppliers)
Bristol House, 40–56 Victoria St, Bristol BS1 6BY
Tel: 0117 929 0661
www.soilassociation.org
E-mail: info@soilassociation.org

OVERSEAS CONTACTS

Australia
Australian Bush Flower Essences
45 Booralie Road, Terrey Hills, NSW 2084
Tel: 02 9450 1388 Fax: 02 9450 2866
www.ausflowers.com.au
E-mail: info@ausflowers.com.au

Australasian College of Natural Therapies
57 Foveaux Street, Surry Hills, NSW 2010
Tel: 02 9218 8850 Fax: 02 9281 4411
E-mail: info@acnt.edu.au

International Federation of Aromatherapists
*To find an IFA accredited aromatherapist in your area call the national information
line:* 01902 240125 *or visit* www.ifa.org.au

Massage Association of Australia

PO Box 1187, Camberwell, Victoria 3124

Tel: 03 9885 7631 Fax: 03 9886 9095

www.maa.org.au

E-mail: info@maa.org.au

Reflexology Association of Australia

PO Box 366, Cammeray, NSW 2062

Tel/Fax: 02 9918 9241

www.raa.inta.net.au

Australian Yoga Masters Association

183 Pitt Town Road, Kenthurst, NSW 2156

New Zealand

New Zealand Natural Health Practitioners Accreditation Board

PO Box 37–491, Auckland

Tel: 09 625 9966

New Zealand Bach Flower Remedies

PO Box 358, Waiuku

Tel/Fax: 09 235 7057

E-mail: bachnz@ps.gen.nz

South Africa

South Africa Homoeopaths, Chiropractors and Allied Professions Board

PO Box 17055, 0027 Groenkloof

Tel: 246 6455

Nutrition Information Centre

Nicus, PO Box 19063, Tygerburg 7505

Tel: 021 933 1408 Fax: 021 933 1405

Index

Piatkus Books

If you have enjoyed reading this book, you may be interested in other titles published by Piatkus. These include:

Acupressure: How to cure common ailments the natural way Michael Reed Gach

Aromatherapy: The encyclopedia of plants and oils and how they help you Danièle Ryman

Beat Stress and Fatigue Patrick Holford

Clear Your Clutter with Feng Shui Karen Kingston

Complete Book of Food Combining, The: Lose weight and feel great with the only guide you'll ever need Kathryn Marsden

Detox Your Mind: Feel the benefits after only 7 days Jane Scrivner

How Meditation Heals: A practical guide to healing your body and your mind Eric Harrison

Little Book of Detox, The: Easy ways to cleanse, revitalise and energise Jane Scrivner

Living Food for Health: 12 Natural Superfoods to transform your health Dr Gillian McKeith

Optimum Nutrition Bible, The Patrick Holford

Optimum Nutrition Cookbook, The Patrick Holford and Judy Ridgway

Perfect Skin: The natural approach Amanda Cochrane

Paitkus Guide to Feng Shui, A Jon Sandifer

Reflexology Handbook, The: A complete guide Laura Norman

Six Weeks to Superhealth: An easy-to-follow programme for total health transformation Patrick Holford

Teach Yourself to Meditate: Over 20 simple exercises for peace, health and clarity of mind Eric Harrison

Vertical Reflexology: A revolutionary five-minute technique to transform your health Lynne Booth

Women's Bodies, Women's Wisdom: The complete guide to women's health and well-being Dr Christian Northrup